Brain Gym
for all
Melodie de Jager

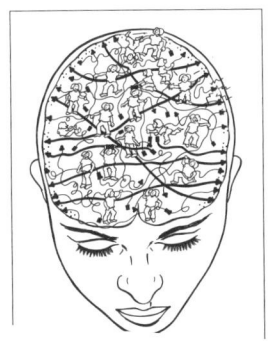

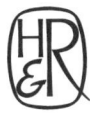

Human & Rousseau
Cape Town Pretoria

Brain Gym® for All was formatted and compiled by
Melodie de Jager based on the collected and original works
of Paul E. Dennison, Carla Hannaford and Gail E. Dennison.

First edition, first impression 2001
Second impression 2001
Third impression 2002
Second edition, first impression 2002
Second impression 2003
Third impression 2004
Third edition, first impression 2005

Copyright © 2001 by Melodie de Jager
Published by Human & Rousseau,
a division of NB Publishers (Pty) Limited,
40 Heerengracht, Cape Town
Cover photograph: Gallo Images/Getty Images
Illustrations by Louwra Marais
Typography by Etienne van Duyker
Cover design by Michiel Botha
Text electronically prepared and set in 11 on 13 pt Janson
by ALINEA STUDIO, Cape Town
Printed and bound by Paarl Print,
Oosterland Street, Paarl, South Africa

ISBN-10: 0-7981-4653-2
ISBN-13: 978-0-7981-4653-1

Dear reader

It would have been great to chat to you about *Brain Gym® for All* over a steaming cup of tea in a room with a view and a crackling fire. But seeing that we can't do that right now, let's talk about the purpose of *Brain Gym® for All*. It has been written as a simple guide for people who would like to be mentally agile and fit. It is not a textbook or a prescription for an instant cure, but an easy read on how to be the best *you* most of the time.

Often people buy books and attend seminars to improve themselves – but *you* don't need improvement. You are perfect just the way you are, with your unique blend of skills and abilities. In this book skills and abilities are described in terms of dominance profiles – giving you a glimpse into survival profiles, which describe a person's behaviour when stressed and as such is a description of the *smallest* number of skills that will ever be available to that person. The profiles aren't the main focus, however. They simply provide a model for shedding some light on why, for instance, your child finds it difficult to sit still and concentrate if he or she doesn't have the opportunity to learn hands-on, or is challenged by suddenly having to copy words correctly or to read accurately. It may even ring a bell about why you need to turn your back on your partner before falling asleep!

These little idiosyncrasies are your personal behavioural signature – which makes you an original and not a copy. You don't want to change that.

So where does *Brain Gym® for All* fit into the picture? You know those moments in life when everything is easy and you feel happy and truly alive? In those moments you are the real *you*. But sometimes, when pressures mount and the expectations of peers, parents, school and employers get too much, you may feel overwhelmed and a little less than yourself. Those are the moments when you seem to lose your footing or feel stuck and unable to produce the goods like you normally do. That's when you need something to get you back on track, and this is where *Brain Gym® for All* comes in.

During my years of being an educator and life coach, the Brain

Gym® movements described in this book have been invaluable tools for kids and adults wanting to give themselves a mental boost when the task or situation demanded it. According to Paul Dennison (the father of Brain Gym®) people love it, request it, teach it to their friends and integrate it into their lives. Some find it helpful over a short period of time to establish a new pattern of behaviour, others may continue using it for a matter of weeks or months to reinforce new learning, and still others may return to their favourite Brain Gym® movements whenever new stresses or challenges crop up.

Brain Gym® is fun and effective – enjoy it!

Melodie

Ps. Should you be interested in more scientific explanations, international research or contact details, kindly refer to the bibliography at the back of the book.

Please note

The movements and activities described in this book are solely for educational purposes. The author does not intend (directly or indirectly) to present any part of this work as a diagnosis or prescription for any condition, nor to make representations concerning the psychological or physical effects of the concepts described in this book. The author is not responsible for anyone misrepresenting this information.

Although these movements and activities have been found to be safe and effective, it is always advisable to consult a medical practitioner before following any movement programme. All the movements are intended to be easy and comfortable to do – it is therefore important to build up skills gradually.

These concepts are not intended to replace any other programme, but can be used to enhance and support all other educational programmes.

Contents

Brain gymnastics?

You can get fit by exercising regularly in a gym or by doing other exercises. Your brain, thoughts, senses and memory can also become **"fit"** if you follow an exercise programme. *Brain Gym® for all* is a personal exercise programme for improved quality of life.

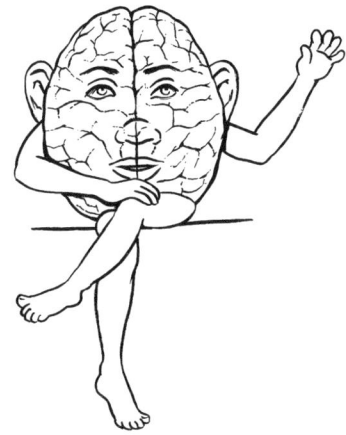

Brain Gym® for all describes a way of life that will help you look to the future with a sense of purpose. We tend to get stuck in certain patterns as far as thinking and behaviour are concerned. Often these patterns are ineffective and do not work **for** you. It doesn't have to be that way: you can change. You can change your thoughts, abilities and skills by doing simple exercises to wake up your brain and alter your thinking patterns. These physical exercises, called Brain Gym®, were originally developed by Dr Paul E. Dennison to help children with learning problems. It was soon realised, however, that these exercises could help to make learning and living easier for **all** people.

When you do Brain Gym® regularly . . .

- stress and anxiety levels drop
- brain integration improves
- performance improves at all levels
- quality of life improves.

People who had to bear the labels of attention deficit disorder, hyper-activity, depression, or underachievement; who were chronically stress-ed and for years suffered from anxiety attacks and poor self-esteem, had good results with Brain Gym® exercises: there was a marked improve-ment after a period of two months of doing the exercises for 15 min-utes every day. Brain Gym® is not a magic cure, however, but a science that has a neuro-chemical basis.

Who started Brain Gym® and why?

In 1969 an American teacher, Dr Paul E. Dennison – who had him-self experienced years of trying to survive the school system as a "learning disabled" child – started conducting intensive research into what happens in the brain during the process of learning.

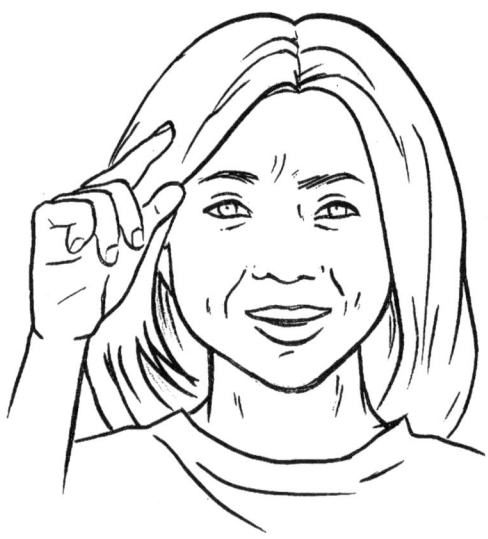

He consulted well-known and respected **sensory-motor experts** such as Drs Doman and Delacato, Jean Ayres, Thomas Tomatis and Newell Kephart, who proved that children can learn anything more easily if their physical development is normal. Dr Dennison also studied the work of Arnold Gesell, Jean Piaget and Maria Montessori, which showed that **abstract concepts** are mastered more easily when they are first experienced in a concrete manner. In addition, he realised anew the importance of each person's **individuality and unique learning style** as described by John Holt, Carl Rogers and Howard Gardener, and, together with this, the implication that people do not all learn in the same way, by sitting still on a chair and listening. He acknowledged the studies of psychologist Alfred Adler and learning expert Spencer Kagan, which proved that people do not function in isolation, but **within a system** and are influenced by the system. Under the guidance of Drs George Goodheart, Sheldon Deal and, in particular, John Thie, he also studied **applied kinesiology** and kinesiology or the **study of movement**, as described by F. Matthias Alexander, Moshe Feldenkrais and Rudolf Laban – all experts in the field of movement.

Dr Dennison's continued, dedicated research into finding techniques to help people learn more easily and effectively, led to Learning Through Movement, or Brain Gym®.

> *Movement is the door to learning. To live is to move. Life is ever changing, ever shifting and ever demanding. Brain Gym teaches us how to move with our challenges, our dreams and our goals. I believe that there are no learning disabilities, only learning blocks. We are all learning blocked to the extent that we have mastered the art of not moving.*
>
> Paul E. Dennison

Brain Gym® for all is a simple self-help guide based on Dr Dennison's research. By setting ourselves goals and carrying out the appropriate **movements**, we can all change old patterns in order to reach new heights in all facets of our lives. The traditional way to tackle learning, life and behavioral problems is through remedial techniques and therapy. *Brain Gym® for all* differs from this traditional approach by focusing more on the **physical** aspects of learning and behaviour, rather than on the cognitive (mental) aspects. Your behaviour and abilities are, to a large extent, determined by the physical functioning of your brain and nervous system. When you revitalise the physical functioning of your brain and nervous system through neurological stimulation, your behaviour and abilities alter, along with your self-image.

9

The key to neurological revitalisation is movement and water.

In *Brain Gym® for all* the value of the following is explored:

- Movement as a natural revitaliser
- The interaction between brain and body
- The brain and body's tendency to specialise and, in so doing, to establish a dominance profile
- Stress and dominance profiles
- The dominance profile as a departure point for change
- A simple model to combat problems and reach new personal and professional heights by:

  ◆ drinking enough water daily
  ◆ setting goals to find direction
  ◆ Brain Gym® as a technique to fine-tune the following abilities:

    ◆ Vision
    ◆ Hearing
    ◆ Eye-hand coordination
    ◆ Reading and spelling
    ◆ Memory
    ◆ Communication
    ◆ Organisation
    ◆ Concentration
    ◆ Combating depression, anxiety and stress.

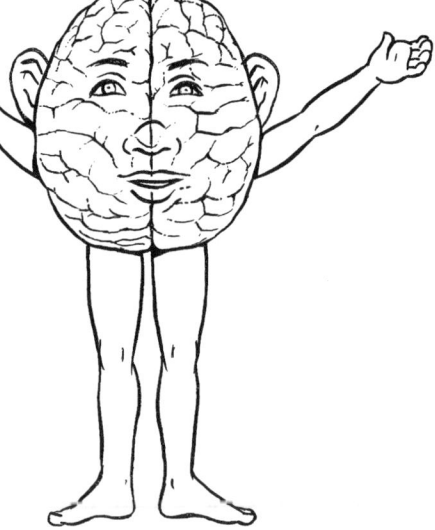

Movement as revitaliser?

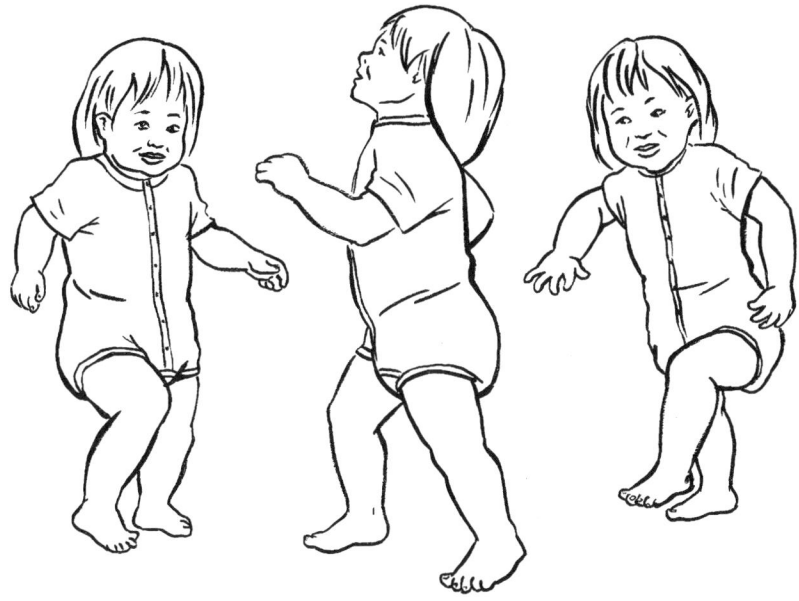

When a person moves (skips, walks, runs or exercises at the gym) their blood circulation is improved throughout the body. Because of the improved circulation and deeper breathing, more oxygen molecules are transported to every cell in the body. The increased oxygen content and polarity in the cell membrane make it easier for messages to move from the senses through the nervous system to the brain. The message is processed in the brain and the brain sends it back to the body through the nervous system, so that one can react.

The moment a baby is born, she starts to move, and as soon as she starts to move, she starts to learn. Faces and smells are soon distinguished so that she can recognise Mom from among many other people.

She also learns that if she cries long and hard enough, she will be picked up, cuddled, changed and possibly fed.

It is estimated that a child acquires half of all the knowledge she will ever learn during the first seven years of life.

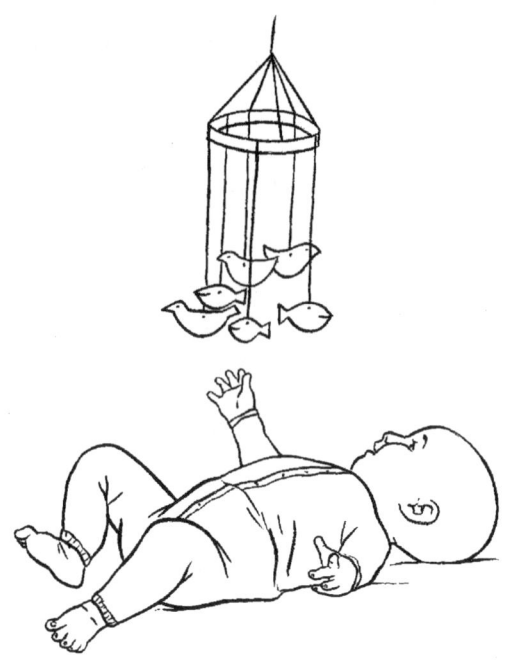

When a baby lies cooing in her cot, her arms and legs seem to move about freely while her head turns towards the colourful mobile. It seems to be a carefree, untrammelled existence, but she is actually hard at work! She is busy doing pioneering work, neurologically speaking, which, in just a few years' time, will enable her to "design" her own picture, read letters, solve problem sums, write poems, play a violin, work out a budget and play a mean game of tennis.

What **determines** a baby's ability to do any of these complex things and what can **prevent** her from doing any of them? It all happens through a network of neurological pathways and connections, and the secretion of important chemicals. The free movements of lifting her head, pressing her knees against her nose, fascination with her hands and rolling around are the beginning of brain integration and physical coordination.

A baby's natural movements and reflexes are developed by a master's hand so that the potential for a happy and successful life lies locked up inside every human being.

The key to unlocking latent potential: MOVEMENT!

As a baby **moves** through all the phases from rolling over to sitting, sitting to crawling, crawling to standing and standing to walking and later running, new neural pathways and connections form between all parts of the brain, as well as between the brain and the body. The baby's constant movement strengthens her muscles and integrates and coordinates all her senses and limbs through a network of neural pathways. By repeating the same thing over and over again, these pathways and networks are established and the basic "wiring" is put in place for later schoolwork, body coordination, personality and behaviour.

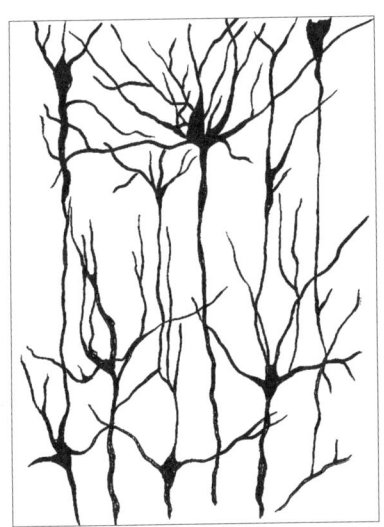 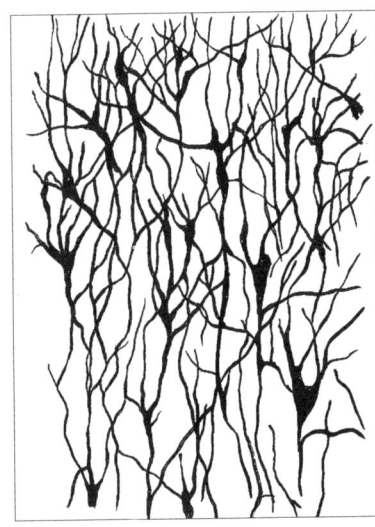

For example, to be able to read in a few years' time, you must have the neural wiring in place so that your eyes can "photograph" the words on a page and reproduce them faithfully, and the image can be sent through the neural pathways to the visual centre in the brain, where the brain interprets the image and gives it meaning. To read aloud from a book is much more difficult, because your hands and eyes must work together and the brain must process messages from your hands and eyes simultaneously, complete the process described above and then, instantaneously, send messages to your speech organs and your ears, so that you can read aloud and also hear yourself.

You are not born with the complete wiring system already connected, but you are born with the potential to be fully connected. The purpose of a baby's developmental stages is to develop and connect the entire body's wiring system through the repetition of the same movements, so that the brain and body can work together effectively. Sometimes . . .

- A child does not complete a developmental stage, such as rolling over, because she seldom lies flat and her days are spent in the supporting "Do-Nut" pillow. When a developmental stage is not completed, the result is underdeveloped networks with weaker connections.

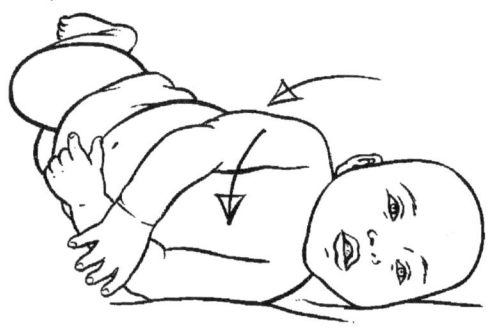

- When a developmental stage, such as crawling, is skipped totally, because the baby slides on her buttocks or is suspended in a walking ring too early, it leads to weaknesses in the neurological structure, almost like a juicy white onion that has one brown layer inside.

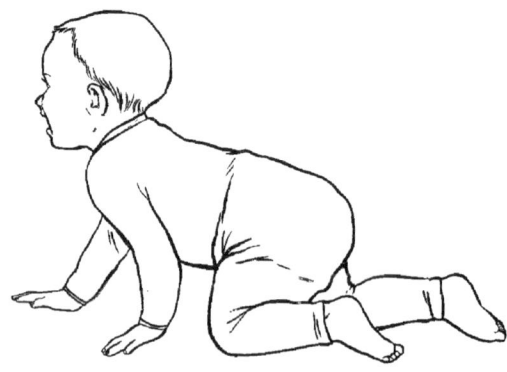

- Stress (biochemical, emotional or physical) and trauma cause some of the existing networks to shut down or get blocked. When someone is traumatised by, for example, a near-drowning, the death of a loved one, illness, an accident, or abuse, existing healthy networks can become blocked and certain functions and abilities, already learned, are, as it were, "lost".

Fragile or blocked networks mean that a person is capable of achieving far more or performing much better than he or she is doing at that moment, but that the underlying connections and wiring are missing. Such a person therefore has far more latent abilities than he realises.

A baby performs somewhere in the region of 50 000 crawling movements in order to integrate the left and right hemispheres of the brain.

What about age?

A lot of people think impaired memory, vision and hearing are simply the natural result of ageing, but research shows that only about 10 percent of your brain cells die during your lifetime. The other 90 percent are still there, ready, willing and able!

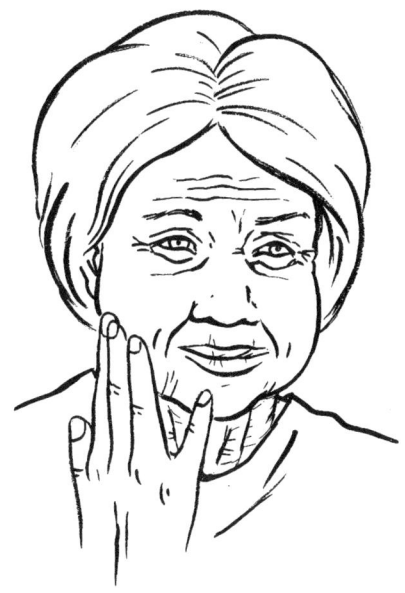

The fact that even the cleverest among us do not even use 7 percent of their brain's capacity leaves a lot of room for improvement.

The good news

Whether developmental stages were either not completed or skipped, or you experienced serious trauma, or you are getting on in years, the ability to form new networks or strengthen existing ones will be there for the rest of your life. The simple Brain Gym® exercises can develop and strengthen networks and keep your brain young and healthy, no matter what age you are.

The interaction between brain and body

Brain Gym® differs from any other learning technique, by focusing on the **physical development** rather than on **mental development**. Research proves that when physical development progresses well, the chances of effective mental development are greater.

Good physical development means that your eyes, ears, hands, feet, the rest of your senses and your entire brain can work together like a well-trained team. If your team functions as a unit, you can probably observe keenly, think, plan, make decisions, explain your decisions, and carry them out.

To demonstrate this process in a practical manner, think about somebody who wants to have a cold drink and listen to music:

Information in
Getting the idea

Processing
Planning

Information out
Carrying out the plan

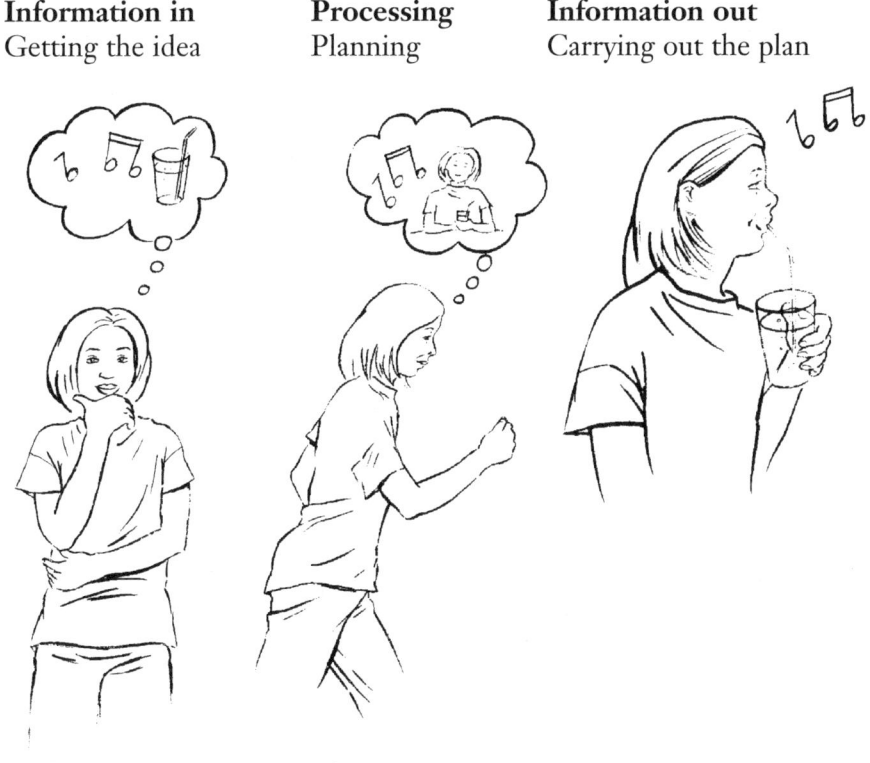

1. Taking in information

Refers to your ability to observe through your senses by:
- smelling and tasting,
- seeing,
- listening,
- feeling (through the skin).

2. Processing information

Refers to your ability to process what you have seen, heard or felt by:
- critical analysis or interpreting the whole,
- thinking about it or getting a feeling about it,
- talking about it or quietly wondering about it.

3. Acting on information

Refers to your ability to react after making a decision by:
- taking action,
- applying the knowledge,
- just knowing it and considering possible actions.

> *Ideally, ALL the senses, parts of the brain and limbs should play together like a symphony orchestra, creating a beautiful, harmonious whole.*

But in reality, all the parts do not always work equally hard together, because you are born with the natural tendency to, for example, use one hand more than the other:

- You always use the same eye to peer through a keyhole.
- There is also the well-known example, which has led to many a fight between couples: your partner thinks you no longer love him because you turn away from him in bed when you want to go to sleep. This is normal and no reflection on your relationship: everybody has a preferred "sleeping side"!

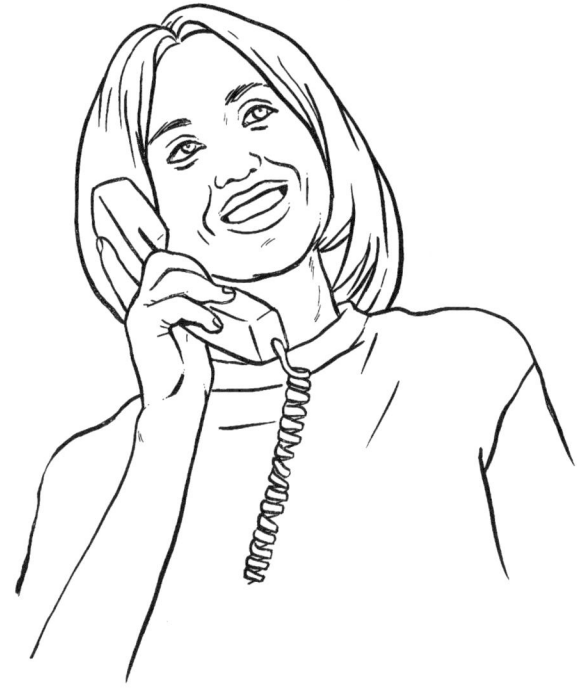

- When you pick up the telephone, you almost always hold it to the same ear. It's only when you have to write something down that you might switch the receiver to the other ear.
- You do not use one hand to sign a cheque today and the other hand tomorrow.

Dominance

As it works in nature, where there are two, one will be the leader.

This does not mean that one will intimidate or overpower the other. Rather, it implies good interaction, as in any healthy relationship: one leads and the other follows and when the situation or context changes, the roles are reversed.

When mother and child cross the street, for example, the mother leads and the child follows.

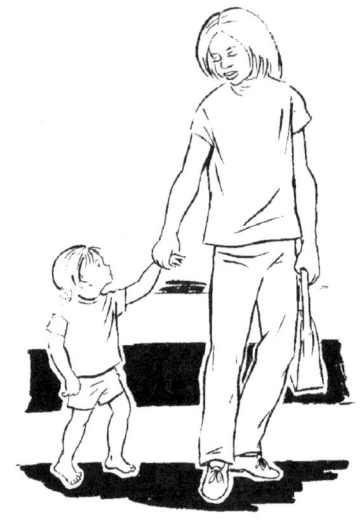

But when they play on the beach, the child can be the leader and the mother follows.

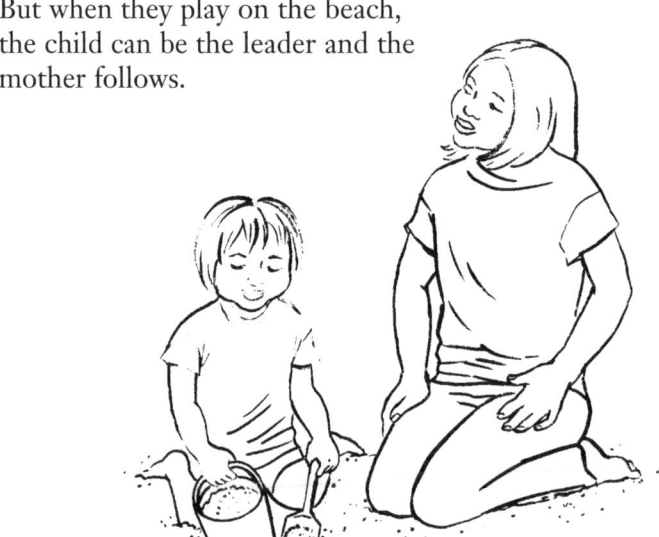

In Brain Gym® dominance means to lead and to specialise. Leading and specialising apply to your senses, limbs and parts of your brain in terms of your own unique way of: .

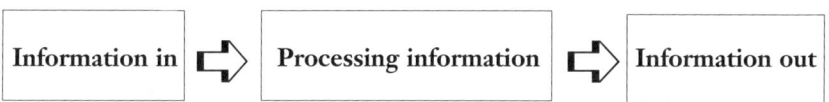

| Information in | ➡ | Processing information | ➡ | Information out |

While conducting his comprehensive research, Dr Dennison realised that every person has a basic specialisation profile – the one you use when your stress levels are going through the roof and the roof tiles come raining down.

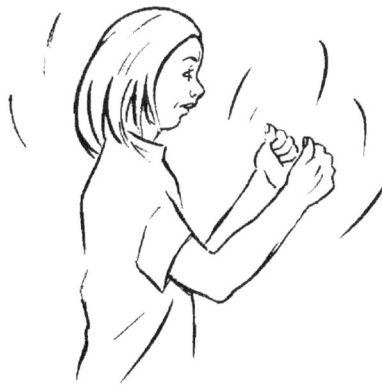

What do you do? Do you run to the telephone and spill out your story into somebody's ear; do you cover your head and cry softly; do you blame the pathetic quality of roof tiles; or do you pick up the tiles and start making a collage around the swimming pool?

Your dominance profile, and thus a specific behaviour code, is genetically determined and influenced by people and circumstances. Ever heard: "That is most definitely a Smith" or "That is the way the Halls do it"? These are inherited, genetically determined behaviour patterns.

Does this mean I am a slave to my dominance profile?

Am I a victim of my ancestry?

Fortunately not . . . but you could be!

21

Remember, you have the ability, throughout your life, to build new neural pathways, which means you can always change **if you want to**. You don't have to be a victim of your ancestry, of badly developed neural networks, too many walking ring escapades, traumatic experiences or depression.

You can change!

The older you are, the stronger the neural pathways that maintain your behaviour pattern and the longer it takes to change the dominance profile.

But it can be done!

The younger you are or your child (whose genetic predisposition doesn't fit in with the teachers' expectations) is, the quicker the networks can be changed because they are not yet firmly entrenched.

Dominance profiles

In order to understand dominance profiles and the effect they have on your behaviour, it might be helpful to look at the history of brain research.

In 1861 Dr Paul Broca, a French doctor, paved the way for research into the differences between the left and right brains. This was the beginning of Cerebral Neurology – a wake-up call to researchers to chart the functions of the brain by studying the effects of brain injury on performance.

The concept of cerebral dominance soon followed, and the human brain was explained in terms of a left and a right brain. Because it was thought that the language area, located in the **left brain** (Broca's Area) is what makes people human, the left brain was also viewed as the dominant brain hemisphere in all people. It was thought that the left brain controlled purposeful movement and clear (articulate) speech.

The **right brain** was seen as less important, with no specific function. Even when research started to indicate that important properties could be assigned to the right brain, the assumption remained that the right brain is the lesser of the two.

It is interesting that, in spite of the latest research (which shows that the right brain is both equal and unique), the academic spotlight still falls on language abilities, and art, music and dancing as learning techniques – and along with them everyone who has a right-brain way of learning – are often belittled.

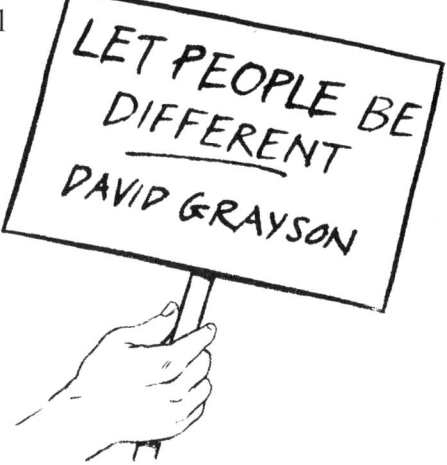

The first commandment of any truly civilised society should be:

People differ, and so do the way they do things, because their dominance profiles differ. When you understand how a dominance profile is put together, you will have a **better understanding** of yourself and others.

What determines a dominance profile?

A dominance profile (as a model of how you function) is determined by many variables. They are called variables because it is the **differing** parts of each person that together make him or her so unique. These variables include your eyes, ears, hands, feet and brain parts as representatives of your ability to take in, process and act on information.

Information in How do you observe?	Information processing How do you process it?	Information out What do you do with it?

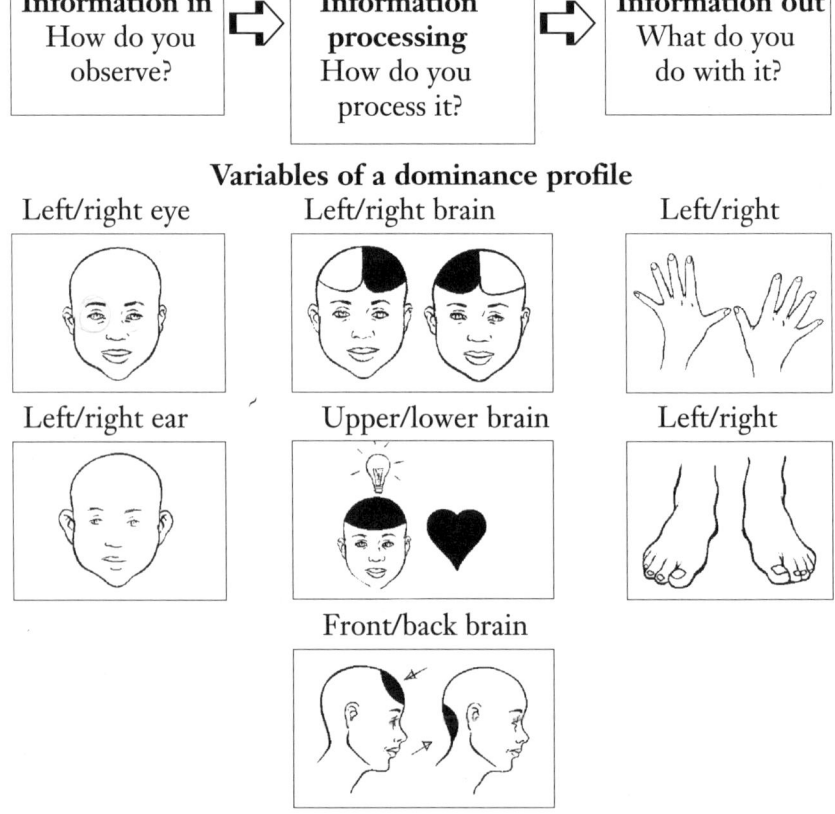

Variables of a dominance profile

Left/right eye   Left/right brain   Left/right

Left/right ear   Upper/lower brain   Left/right

Front/back brain

All these variables are put together in a diagram so that the mutual interactions can be observed and interpreted.

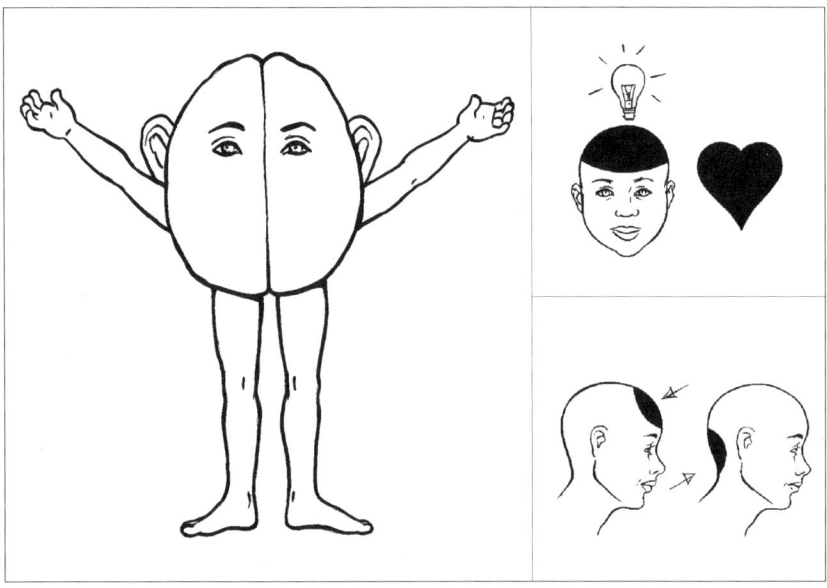

A complete and responsible interpretation of a dominance profile is complex and for this reason the services of a qualified Brain Gym® consultant are recommended. But if, out of interest, you would like to make your own interpretation, complete the following questionnaire.

How do I determine my dominance ?

Dominance test

Circle each appropriate answer on the right:

EYE	Wink – which eye is open?	L	R
	Aim – which eye is open?	L	R
	Kaleidoscope – which eye looks through the hole at the colours and patterns?	L	R
EAR	Hold a shell to your ear.	L	R
	Answer the telephone.	L	R
HAND	Your writing hand.	L	R
	In which hand do you hold your knife?	L	R
	Which hand opens lids?	L	R
FOOT	Which foot do you use to kick?	L	R
	Which foot takes the first step on a high step?	L	R

Circle the words in the right-hand column if the statement is true for you:

THE BRAIN		
LEFT/ RIGHT	When reading, do you prefer words only on the page?	Left
	Or do you like pictures in between?	Right
	Are you creative?	Right
	Are you very neat and tidy?	Left
	Do you like change?	Right
	Do you like drawing up lists?	Left
FRONT/ BACK	Are you quiet at social gatherings?	Back
	Do you find it easy to make contact with strangers?	Front
	Do you treasure your time alone?	Back
	Do you prefer being among people?	Front
	Do you like taking the lead?	Front
	Do you like supporting other people?	Back
UPPER/ LOWER	Do you ever say: I **think** we should . . . ?	Top
	Do you perhaps say: I **feel** it would be nice if . . . ?	Bottom
	Do people say to you: Stop **feeling** and **think** for a change ?	Bottom

Colour in your dominant variables on the diagram below.

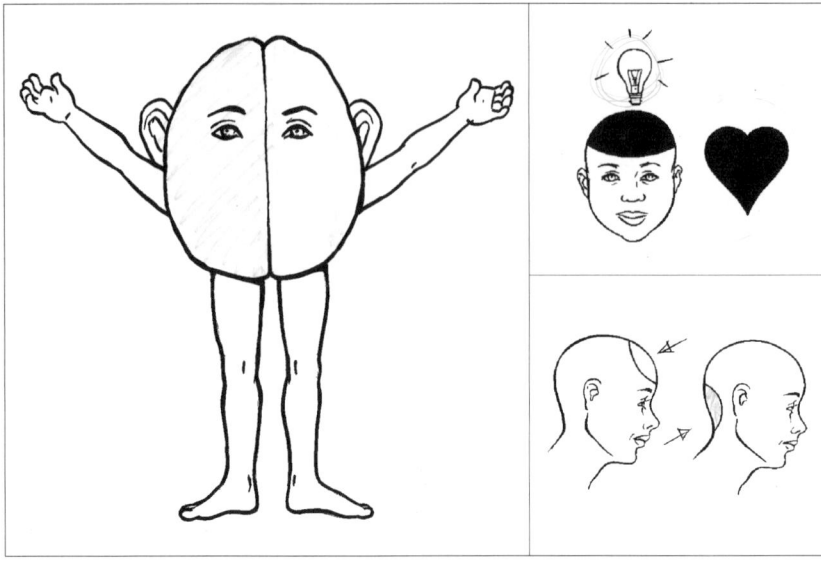

Many people will, on their own, notice very little difference between the variables, and might be tempted to circle everything. This indicates good integration and development as a person. In psychology, such a person is referred to as *mature*.

After determining your profile, ask someone who knows you well to fill in the questionnaire on your behalf, as they see you. Compare the two to find out if other people see you in the same way as you see yourself.

What do the variables mean?

To interpret your dominance profile, you have to pay attention to the variables and their meanings. The ideal would be to use your entire brain and all your senses simultaneously to observe. But the volume of information that is there to be observed at any one time is overwhelming, so your brain chooses to sift through the information and pay attention to certain aspects only. Your dominance profile indicates the way you sift information, which implies that a lot of information is left out.

All dominance profiles are valuable and suited to specific tasks, but because information is ignored, some profiles are more suitable for certain situations and tasks than others. It would provide great insight if you could get an idea of what your brain instinctively pays attention to and what it instinctively ignores. This natural and unconscious sifting process has a direct impact on the way you learn and live. It highlights your strong and weaker characteristics, so that you can, perhaps, understand why you tend to take over in a new situation, or keep to yourself; why, two days after an argument that left you speechless, you have no trouble coming up with brilliant rejoinders; and why you like reading, or prefer not to read.

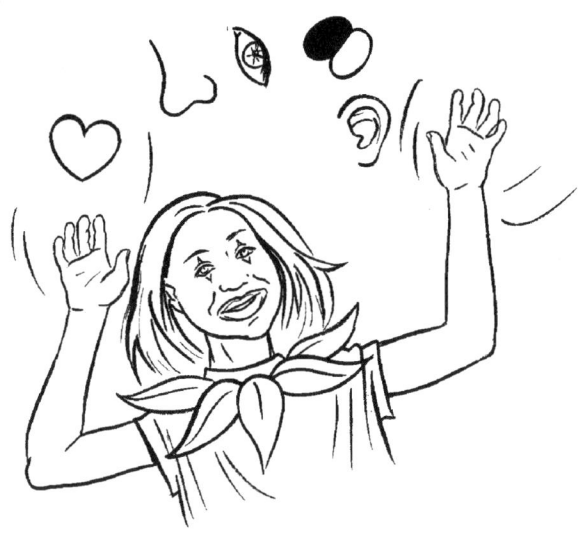

To interpret your dominance profile, you must remember that the right side of your body is controlled and managed by your left brain. The left side of your body is controlled and managed by your right brain. The functions of your senses and limbs will thus correspond to the functions and characteristics of the controlling brain hemisphere. We shall ignore tasting and smelling for now, because **seeing, hearing** and **feeling** are the most common "learning senses".

Keep your dominance profile diagram close at hand so that you can use it as a model for the unique way in which you sift information. The dominant variables in the diagram are your model for how you observe, process and react. The non-dominant variables give you an idea of which options you instinctively ignore when you observe, process and react.

1. Information in

The ears

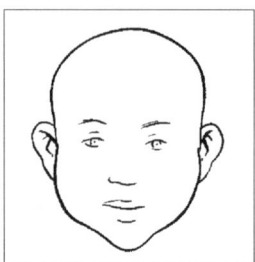

Your ears listen in completely different ways and pay attention to different facets of what is being heard. Check which ear was marked dominant in your diagram – left or right. The following characteristics describe how you listen:

Left ear listens:
- creatively
- to intonation
- to *how* something is said
- emotionally
- subjectively
- far and wide, and hears everything
- with intuitive empathy

- and generalises information

- to the story
- to understand

Right ear listens:
- logically
- analytically
- to *what* is being said
- systematically, point by point
- objectively
- focused

- to word order and sentence construction
- to the information and breaks it down into smaller parts
- to the facts
- to remember

The eyes

As with your ears, the functions of your eyes differ. The right eye sees things more realistically (as they are) and correctly, while the left eye sees more idealistically and hopefully (as they could be). This also explains why the right eye reads more easily than the left eye – the right eye sees the words as they are, but the left eye scans and interprets what is being read. For this reason the left eye prefers a book with pictures and "reads" the pictures, rather than the words; it easily reads "home" instead of "house".

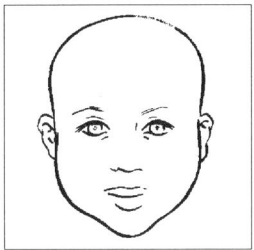

Left eye:
- reads from right to left
- doesn't like many words and therefore doesn't like reading
- looks at the whole
- looks at the big picture
- looks at the meaning
- looks creatively at what **could be**
- looks at colour and form
- focuses more easily on distance than nearby on a book

Right eye:
- reads from left to right
- devours words and numbers and therefore likes reading
- analyses
- looks at the detail
- looks for accuracy
- looks critically at what **is**
- looks at line and symmetry
- focuses more easily nearby on a book than on distance

2. Processing

Parts of the brain

The brain is divided into three dimensions, each with two opposites:

- **Left** (logical and verbal)/**Right** (global and creative)
- **Front** (expressive and extrovert)/**Back** (receptive and introvert)
- **Upper** (cognitive/thinking)/**Lower** (emotional/affective)

As with your senses and limbs, you also have a dominant brain part in each dimension that determines how you think and plan.

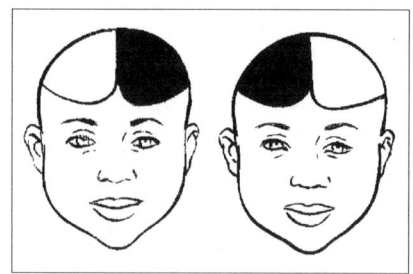

The left brain:
- is logical and verbal
- communicates with words
- is goal-oriented
- is analytical
- has a good concept of time
- is future-oriented
- is ordered
- is task-oriented
- is compulsive
- controls emotions, hides feelings

The right brain:
- is global/overall and creative
- communicates with gestures and body language
- is experience-oriented
- creates synthesis
- has a loose concept of time
- is "now"-oriented
- likes free association
- is people-oriented
- is impulsive
- is emotionally spontaneous, shows feelings

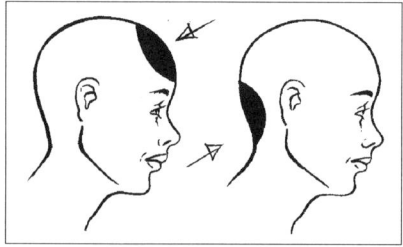

The front brain:
- is expressive
- is action driven
- is focused
- is active
- is proactive
- is more like an extrovert
- is externally oriented – interpersonal

The back brain:
- is receptive
- is thoughtful
- is intuitive
- is passive
- is reactive
- is more like an introvert
- is internally oriented – intrapersonal

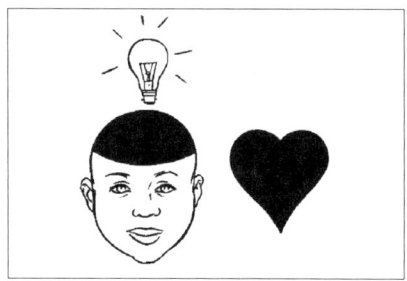

The upper brain:
- is cognitive (thinking)
- is rational
- is retentive/conservative/good
- is reserved
- is sharp and to the point
- is unemotional
- is neat and orderly

The lower brain:
- is affective (feeling)
- is irrational
- is impulsive
- is passionate
- is woolly and vague
- is emotional
- homely, likes atmosphere

3. Information out

The hands

Your hands symbolise the way you communicate – how you speak and write. Left-handed people gesticulate freely (ever seen a left-handed person give directions over the phone?), speak and write in similes and metaphors. Right-handed people are more precise when they communicate: "On 31 March 2000 there were 29 winners in the state lottery, who each won R2 300 246,00", as opposed to the left-handers': "Wow, that bunch of people won millions!" Right-handed people tend to write neatly and correctly on the lines, while left-handed people prefer to draw, build or make shapes. They are thus more skilled manually than verbally.

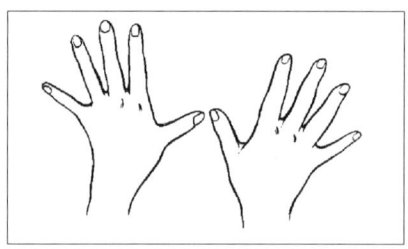

Left hand prefers:
- free movement
- bold, fluent writing
- a creative writing style
- figures of speech, emotion and meaning
- unlined paper
- drawing and touching
- to supplement language with gestures

Right hand prefers:
- fine motor movements
- neat and precise writing
- a structured writing style
- attention to syntax and semantics
- lined paper
- writing
- an extensive vocabulary and is well spoken

The feet

The feet symbolise the way you move (large motor movements) and how you handle new situations and challenges. The right foot (controlled by the left brain) is precise and consistent in its movement, which is obvious in athletes competing in high jump, long jump and hurdles – "right-footers" always keep in step. The pace of "left-footers" tends to vary and they cannot always keep in step.

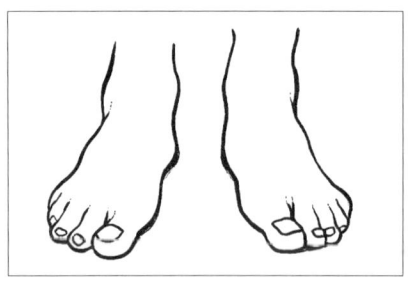

Left foot likes:	**Right foot likes:**
• freedom of movement	• precise and controlled movement
• giant leaps	• controlled and accurate actions
• variety and change	• consistency
• impulsive actions	• a conservative approach
• fluidity of movement	• technique

When you put together the meaning of all the variables, you will see that there is a lot of information. Many of the characteristics and functions may seem contradictory. If a characteristic appears more than once in the different variables, there is a good chance that this specific characteristic has a strong neural network and you are thus very skilled at it. If, for example, you have a left-, upper- and front-brain dominance you are definitely a brilliant thinker, planner and doer. On the other hand, if you have a right-, back- and lower-brain dominance, you are without doubt a passionate and creative individual.

The purpose of dominance profiles

The purpose of a dominance profile is to **understand** why you sometimes act as you do and have difficulty performing certain tasks. If all the **variables** are processed statistically, you will find that there are 196 possible dominance profiles and just as many types of people!

The primary purpose of dominance profiles is thus to realise that people are **different** in themselves, and in the way they observe and experience things. For this reason, other people are not headstrong or stubborn . . .

They are simply wired that way.

Your boss is not an insensitive monster if he says: "Yes, that's all very well, but please get to the point." And you are not undisciplined or incoherent if you give a lot more information than is relevant; it may just be that you experience things within a broader framework and the framework is essential to the story.

People differ and because they differ they also learn differently and experience the same situations differently – which makes it tricky to find the **truth**: whose is the real truth? For each person it is his or her own . . .

But do not fall into the trap of viewing your profile as limiting. Your dominance profile is simply a **tendency profile**, not who you are. You are much more than just a left or right brain! At the very most, your profile can only give you an indication of how you might react in a stressful situation and how other people might interpret your behaviour.

Each profile has its advantages and disadvantages. The advantages of your dominance profile are the characteristics you **have and use** for quality of life. The disadvantages are the characteristics you **unconsciously ignore**, which are therefore not as easy to use and experience in your day-to-day life.

The complexity of dominance profiles makes their interpretation difficult, which is why this is a specialised field. Consulting a qualified Brain Gym® consultant is still recommended for a complete and responsible interpretation of dominance profiles.

Stress and dominance profiles

Our modern lifestyle provides the ideal breeding ground for stress and burnout. It is a continuous rat race to provide for our basic needs, keep appointments, prepare for examinations and presentations, doing a hundred and one things simultaneously and in the end still get good marks or deliver good-quality work.

When you are relaxed, there is a continuous flow of vitality and energy through your body and you can live up to your maximum potential. You secrete endorphins which make you feel good and stimulate your immune system. But when your body experiences stress, your brain divides the available energy to focus on the part experiencing the stress and a part of your brain power is redeployed – away from the brain.

When you are stressed, your survival instinct is activated to fight the threat, by fighting, fleeing or freezing. Your survival instinct and intense experiences of anxiety, worry, fear and depression send high-priority messages to the body to be ready for action:

- Your muscles shorten to strengthen your body,
- Your eyes and ears observe over the full 360 degrees to establish from which direction the "attack" will come,
- Your skin pales because blood rich in oxygen flows to the muscles – away from the thinking centres of your brain,
- Your breathing becomes shallower,
- Adrenaline starts pumping.

It is very difficult to learn and work in a constantly stressful atmosphere, because you battle to concentrate; struggle to think logically and rationally; your memory switches off so that you can concentrate on the present situation; original and creative ideas are inhibited; and you function from your basic dominance profile.

Your basic dominance profile may be excellent for social situations, but it is not necessarily appropriate to the normal life of going to school, studying and going to work. Should your basic dominance profile gain the ascendancy here too, it could become impossible (just as it is for many other people with different profiles) to work and study. This does not mean that there is something wrong with you, just that your "wiring" is different, and you learn just as successfully as anyone else; but the method has to change.

If it is just you or your child who struggle to perform, one can go to the individual to find the "fault". As about 60 percent of people underachieve academically, one could perhaps look at the institution and presentation methods as well. If someone masters the work with enthusiasm and ease with one teacher or facilitator but doesn't get there with another, it is quite possible that his profile and the "good" teacher or facilitator's profile supplement each other and for this reason he can learn. He did not change – the method did!

Does this mean that there have to be as many teaching methods (at least 196) as there are possible dominance profiles to give all the learners an equal opportunity? No . . .

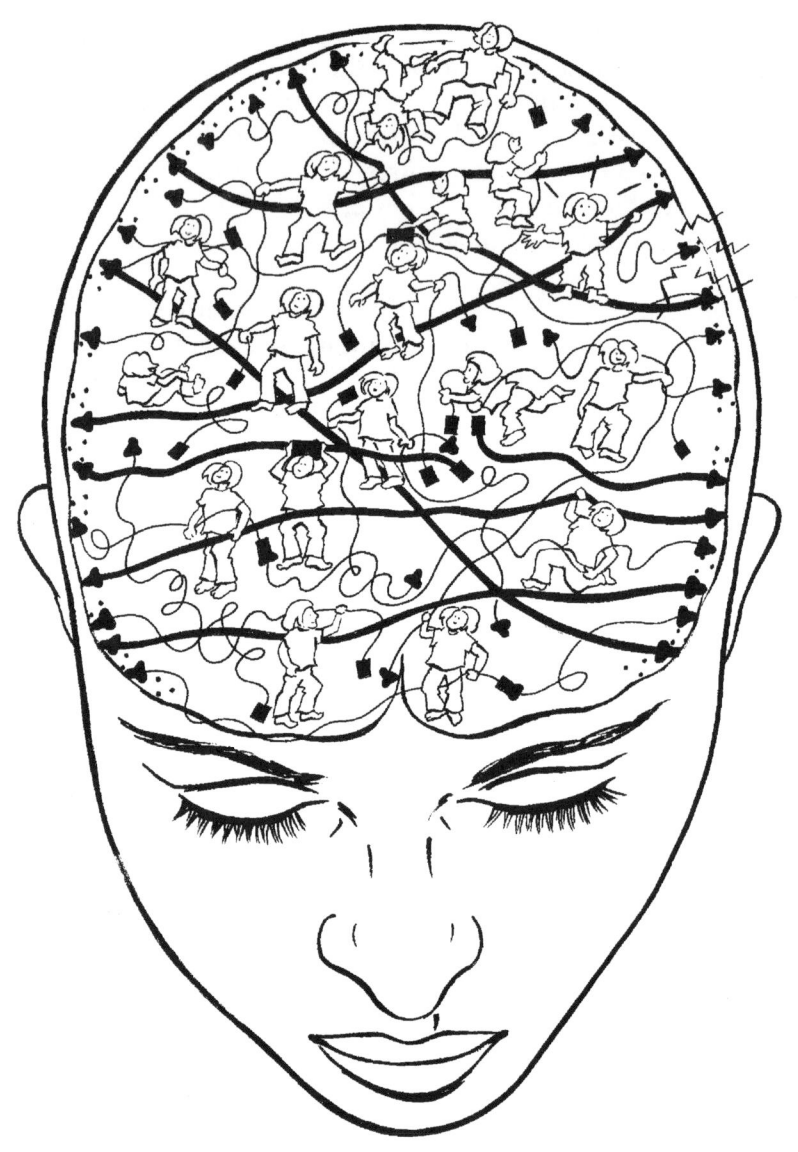

"Rewire" him with Brain Gym®!

A possible solution

It is practically impossible to accommodate all learners' preferences in a large group. The most practical approach is to ensure that all learners learn equally easily using their whole brain and all their senses; then the presentation method becomes irrelevant. In this way, everybody can learn equally effectively, at the same time, with the same teacher or facilitator.

Brain Gym® was developed to build and strengthen neural pathways between **all** your senses and **all** parts of your brain by the repetition of easy, fun exercises. Your skills and behaviour options will more than double if all your variables are working together.

The whole is more than the sum of the parts.

- When you start using both your hands instead of overworking your right hand, your stress levels will be reduced and you will experience less muscle tension in your neck and shoulders.
- Deteriorating eyesight can be the result of underused ears; if you stimulate your hearing, your eyes are able to relax more.
- Your pessimism and negativity could be the result of a well-developed left brain, which is logical and critical by nature. By stimulating the creative and emotional parts of your brain, you can become more positive, optimistic and hopeful and in this way add a new dimension to interpersonal relationships.
- Your inability to be on time, maintain order and remember the dog food, could be the result of a well-developed creative right brain; by stimulating the left (logical) brain, you might even be able to finish those long-postponed projects!

Brain Gym®

By following *Brain Gym® for all*'s four-step programme you will strengthen strong points and stimulate nondominant parts to bring all your latent abilities to the fore. This is the starting point for personal and professional growth on the road to excellence, relaxation and success.

- **Step 1**   **Water as the source of life**

- **Step 2**   **Setting goals**

- **Step 3**   **Specific Brain Gym® exercises**

- **Step 4**   **Neurological maintenance**

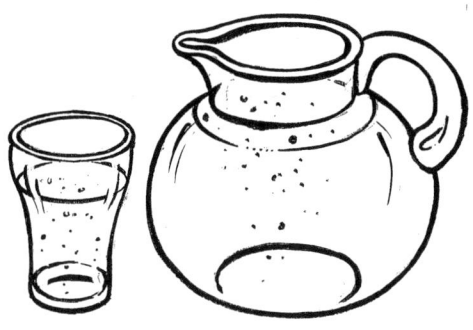

Step 1: Water

Starting today, drink a glass of water instead of coffee, tea or cold drinks during one of your breaks. Your body consists of about 75 percent water and your brain of about 90 percent. When you drink too little water, a high concentration of waste products builds up in your bloodstream and your blood carries less oxygen and nutrients to your cells. The result is weaker cells, which are more susceptible to disease, and make the learning process, in particular, more difficult.

Water aids the solution of minerals in your body, forming electrolytes that charge the cells positively inside and negatively outside. These positive and negative cell charges form the basis of your body's energy. Your brain is the dynamo that generates the electricity or body energy and spreads it throughout your body with the help of the nervous system. To maintain electrical balance in your brain, you need balanced cell charges and sufficient water in your system.

When you get dehydrated, you cannot think clearly and quickly, learn and remember.

Coffee, tea, your favourite tipple and Oros do not count as water, although they contain a lot of water. The body identifies such fluids as food with the result that the breaking-down process is much slower and it takes much longer to isolate the water that dissolves the salts needed for balanced cell charges and a good energy flow.

When you are stressed, high doses of adrenaline are released which enable you to react strongly and swiftly. Recent research shows that the release of adrenaline goes hand in hand with that of another chemical, cortisol, which is known to inhibit the ability to learn and remember. The result of too little water and too much adrenaline and cortisol is an extremely irritable individual who cannot sit still, concentrate or learn.

You need to drink at least **four glasses of water per day** to reduce the effects of stress and maintain balanced, consistent energy levels.

Step 2: Goal

With enough water in your system, you are like a car that's full of fuel and ready to go. **But where to? What is the goal? What do you want to achieve?**

Just like a computer, your brain has many programmes with file names such as: "I am hopeless" or "I am clever" or perhaps "I cannot spell". Some files add positive value to your life, but there are always a few that are negative or confining. These are the ones that grip you and hold you back so that you cannot live life to the fullest. They are the files that, just like a mole, undermine all your good intentions. But fortunately, just as you can delete or edit computer files, you can delete or edit your negative and confining files using a technique like Brain Gym®.

First you have to retrieve the old file.

To be able to delete or edit a file, you first have to retrieve it. So take some time to think about how easy or difficult it is for you to learn; your sense of order; your planning; working and relaxing; your relationships – familial and social; and your emotions. Do you feel happy, content and fulfilled? In which area of your life is there something that causes you trouble and makes you angry? Decide which characteristic, attitude or behaviour you would like to change. It can be absolutely anything.

If you can dream it, you can do it.

Think of a few goals and write them down:

— to concentrate completely while drawing -
— to stop be relashig agresive laughp
for le past & projecting them on
le future

Test your most important goal by asking the following questions:

- Does the goal concern you or is it for somebody else? Remember: you have control over your own behaviour only and can therefore

42

only set goals for **yourself**. Goals such as the following do not concern you: "Mary is less arrogant" or "Shaun does his own homework". Rephrase a new goal that is directed at you, e.g. "I am patient with Mary and Shaun" or "I have self-confidence" or "I wash dishes with enthusiasm" or "I am more positive about the future". Fix the "dripping tap" today.

- Is your goal positive? Does your sentence contain a **not**? "I do **not** want to be shy" or "I do **not** want to be depressed".

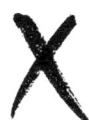 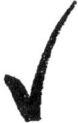

I do not want to be shy	I have self-confidence
I do not want to be depressed	I am happy and energetic
I cannot spell	I can spell
I do not want to go to school	I make school an adventure

Step 3: Brain Gym®

Choose one of the groups of Brain Gym® exercises that can edit your file and rewire your brain so you can reach your goal. The Brain Gym® exercises grouped for specific goals are described fully, in alphabetical order, in Chapter 17 on pages 80-96.

Step 4: Maintenance

Do the exercises every day and remember why you are doing them: What is your goal?

Brain Gym® exercises work whether you have a goal or not.

But your goal is a means to measure your growth and change.

Initially the exercises might be difficult because of badly developed or damaged networks, but they become easier with repetition. In the beginning you are **building** neural pathways and with daily repetition of your set of exercises you are **using** the new pathways that provide easy access to your new or edited file.

Research has proved that change can be permanent as a result of the **intensity** of an experience or of its **repetition**. In *Brain Gym® for all* we use both techniques to ensure fast, permanent change.

At the start of each group of exercises there is an easy test for you to do so that you can compare your performance before and after doing the Brain Gym® exercises. This comparison, as well as the improvement that is often immediately visible, is an excellent motivation to continue exercising.

Brain Gym® is safe – it cannot harm you!

Start at Step 1 (drink water) and do each exercise **slowly**; the slower the better. Stay within your current limits without forcing yourself, and work gradually towards doing more repetitions. According to research, three repetitions of each exercise are sufficient to stimulate a new neural pathway.

Each person's problem is unique and so is its solution. It remains the best option to consult a Brain Gym® consultant, who can determine the right combination of exercises to give you the quickest and most effective results. If there is no Brain Gym® consultant in your area, *Brain Gym® for all* is your answer. The exercise programmes contained in this book are not the only effective combinations: they were grouped together because, in practice, they were shown to be the best for the specific goals. These are recommendations, but any combination or even all the exercises, can be done every day.

You cannot do too many!

Brain Gym® for better vision

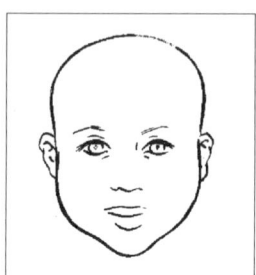

The eyes look, but the brain sees. Your eyes look and the images you see turn upside down and back to front while they move via the optic nerve to the occipital lobes at the back of the brain. As soon as the images reach the occipital lobes, your memory is awakened. What you see now is associated with what you have seen, heard, felt, tasted or smelt before, and thus gets meaning.

Your eyes must work together well if you are to form a clear, life-like picture in your brain. Each eye perceives the same object in a different way and when the different pictures are overlapped in the brain, they should supplement one another. When your eyes are not working together, the picture in your brain can be confusing, not make sense and so make reading difficult. For good interaction it is important for both eyes to move together well. Test how your eyes interact:

Pretest

Hold your head up straight and note how your eyes feel when you do the following:

✔Move your eyes from left to right, following the ceiling.
✔Move your eyes from left to right, from ear to ear.

✔Focus on the floor and move your eyes from left to right.
✔Hold your thumb at a comfortable distance from your eyes and follow your thumb from left to right.

Do your eyes feel equally comfortable with all four tests, or do they burn or feel jumpy?

Brain Gym®

Do the following Brain Gym® exercises **slowly**.

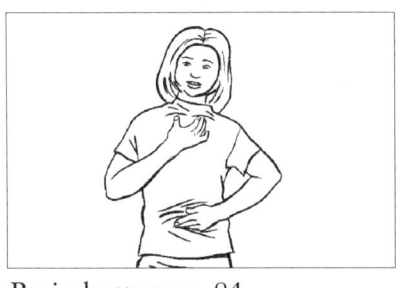
Brain buttons p. 84

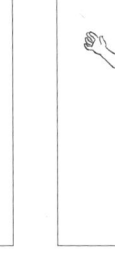
Cross-crawl p. 86

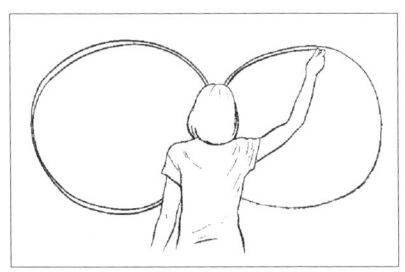
Lazy-8 p. 92

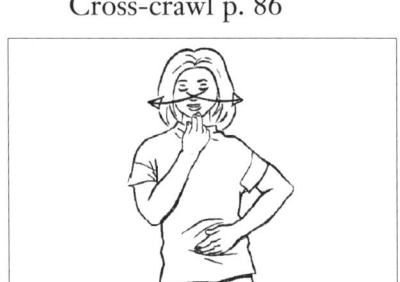
Earth buttons p. 87

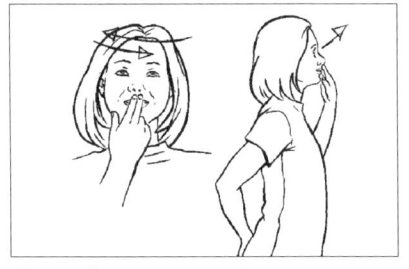
Space buttons p. 95

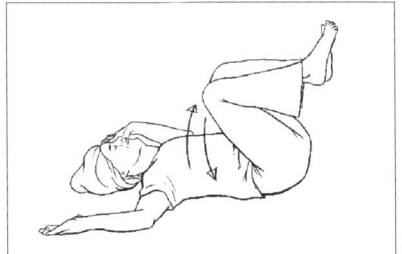
Rocker p. 95

Posttest

How is your sight, and how do your eyes feel now when making the following movements?
✔Move your eyes from left to right, following the ceiling.
✔Move your eyes from left to right, at ear height.
✔Focus on the floor and move your eyes from left to right.
✔Hold your thumb at a comfortable distance from your eyes and follow your thumb from left to right.

Do your eyes feel equally comfortable with all four tests, or do your eyes still burn or feel jumpy?

Brain Gym® for effective listening

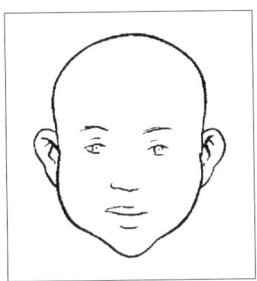

To listen effectively with both ears, your "receptors" must be well developed. The pinna or outer ear is the receiving apparatus of your hearing and absorbs all the sound frequencies in the air. Tiny hairs in the inner ear convert them into sound impulses to which the brain can assign meaning.

The Brain Gym® exercises for effective listening strengthen the neural pathways from the outer ear to the brain and from the brain to the hands, legs and speech organs so that you can listen **and** react.

Pretest

✔Turn your head to the left as far as you can, trying to look behind you.

✔Turn your head to the right as far as you can, trying to look behind you.

✔Turn your head from side to side while you hum aloud. Listen to your voice. Do both ears hear equally clearly, or is one less clear?

Brain Gym®

Do the following Brain Gym® exercises **slowly**.

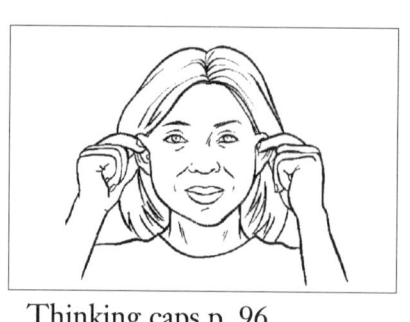

Thinking caps p. 96

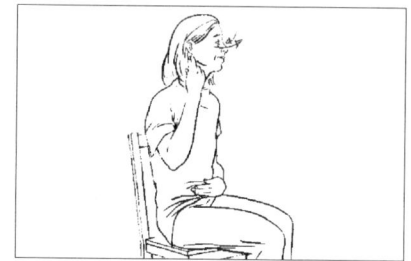

Owl p. 94

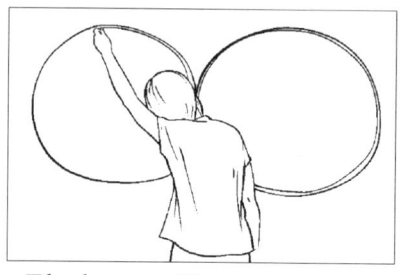

Elephant p. 88

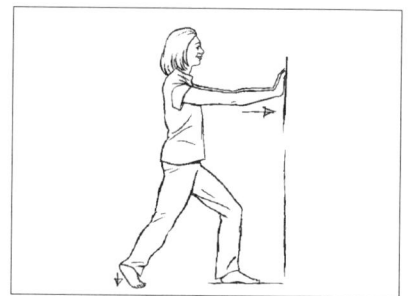

Balance buttons p. 82

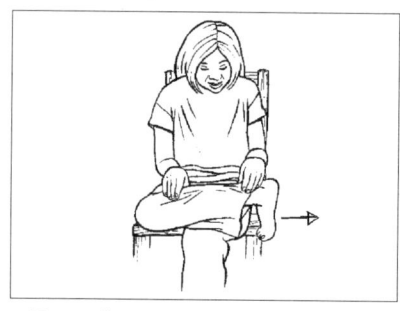

Foot flex p. 89

Calf pump p. 85

Posttest

Test your hearing again:
- ✔ Turn your head to the left as far as you can, trying to look behind you.
- ✔ Turn your head to the right as far as you can, trying to look behind you.
- ✔ Turn your head from side to side while you hum aloud. Listen to your voice. Do both ears hear equally clearly, or is one still not clear?

Brain Gym® for clear and fluent writing

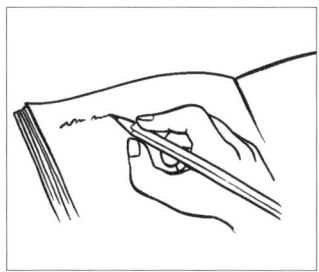

Clear, fluent writing is the result of good fine-motor control – needed for writing, cutting and picking up objects. It is only possible if the large-muscle groups are well developed, enabling you to sit up straight, keep your head upright and move your arms freely.

A strict nursery school teacher who expects youngsters to colour inside the lines too early, or a primary school teacher who insists, too soon, on small, neat writing between the lines, can unconsciously cause a lot of stress when it comes to writing. For this reason, the Brain Gym® exercises start out with big, free-flowing movements to create a positive association with writing. All these writing exercises should preferably be done at eye level, using thick crayons, on an opened-out sheet of newspaper. Neatness is not a factor!

Pretest

✔ Hold a pen and pay attention to your grip. Is it easy and relaxed or does your nail colour change because you put too much pressure on the pen?
✔ Hold a pencil or crayon and pay attention to your grip. Is it the same as for the pen or is it different?
✔ Write down your goal and pay attention to the comfort/discomfort with which you write.

Brain Gym®

Do the following Brain Gym® exercises **slowly**.

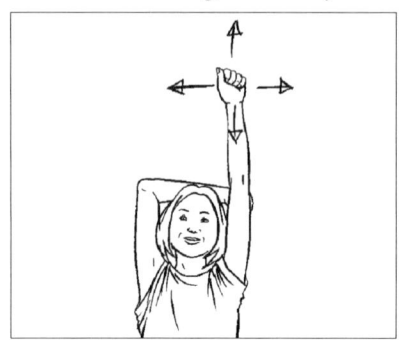

Arm activation p. 81

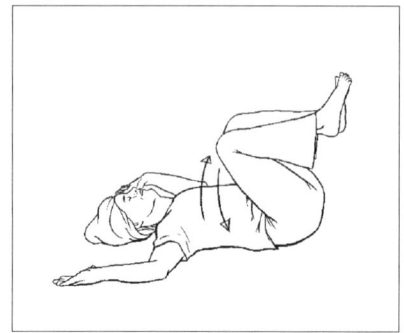

Rocker p. 95

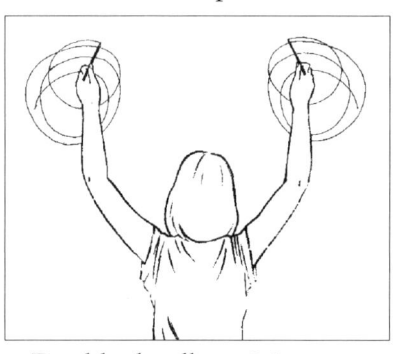

Double doodle p. 86

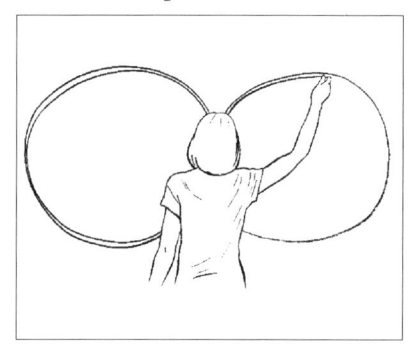

Lazy-8 p. 92

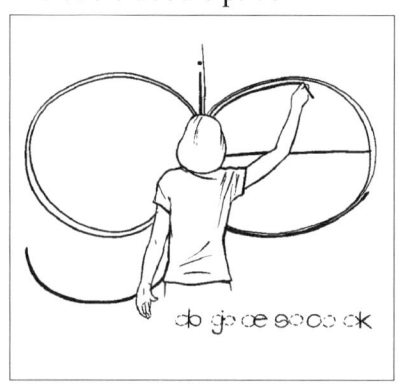

Alphabet-8 p. 80

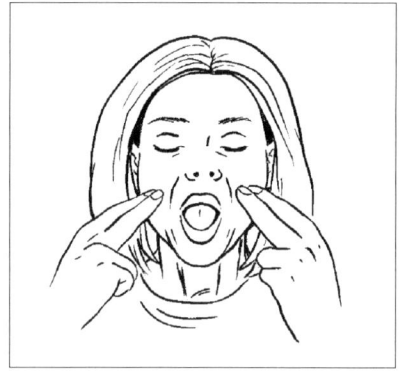

Energy yawn p. 89

Posttest

Test the grip on your pen and writing fluency:

✔Hold a pen and pay attention to your grip. Is it easy and relaxed or does your nail colour change because you put too much pressure on the pen?

✔Hold a pencil or crayon and pay attention to your grip. Is it the same as for the pen or is it different?

✔Write down your goal and pay attention to the comfort/discomfort with which you write.

Brain Gym® for reading and correct spelling

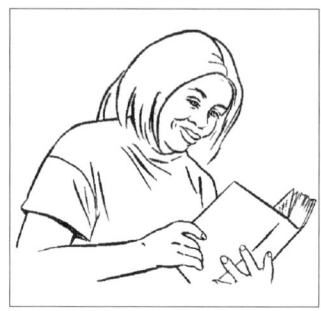

Your dominant eye determines **how** (in what way) and to **what** you will pay attention with your eyes. If your **left eye** (right-eye field) is dominant, your eyes naturally track from **right to left**, which can lead to reversals and spelling problems. Do you page through magazines from front to back or from back to front? If you page from front to back, your right eye (left-eye field) is probably dominant and if you page from back to front, your left eye (right-eye field) is dominant.

Right-eye dominance is an advantage in the Western world, where we read and write from left to right, because the **right eye** naturally tracks from **left to right**. But irrespective of which eye is dominant, good cooperation from both eyes is needed if you are to see, read and spell easily. Your eyes must be able to move together comfortably from left to right, without burning. Your dominance may be fixed, but with exercise the right eye can learn to lead and the left eye to follow. So a left-eye dominance is not the end of the world.

Pretest

✔Read a paragraph. How much can you remember of what you read?

- ✔Read another piece aloud and listen to your voice. What does it sound like?
- ✔Does your head move when you read, or is it stationary?
- ✔Recall a difficult word you have read before. Look up. Can you see the word clearly in your mind's eye?

Brain Gym®

Do the following Brain Gym® exercises **slowly** to strengthen your "wiring" for good reading and spelling.

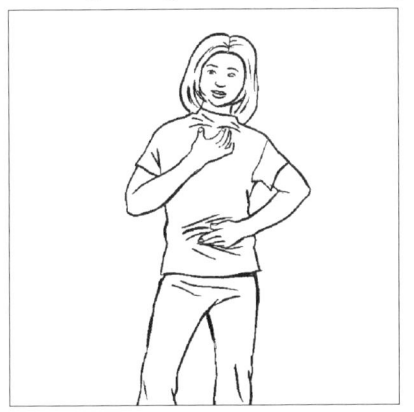

Brain buttons p. 84

Cross-crawl p. 86

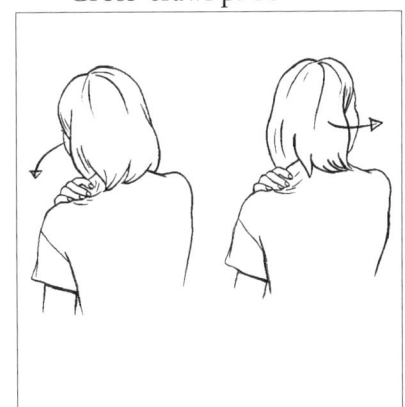

Thinking caps p. 96

Owl p. 94

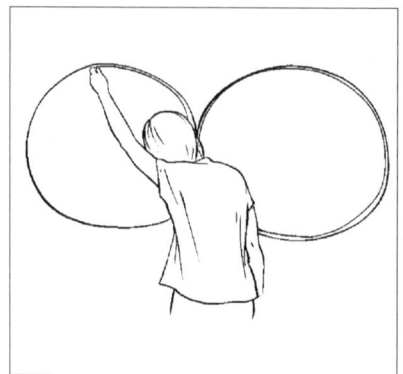

Elephant p. 88

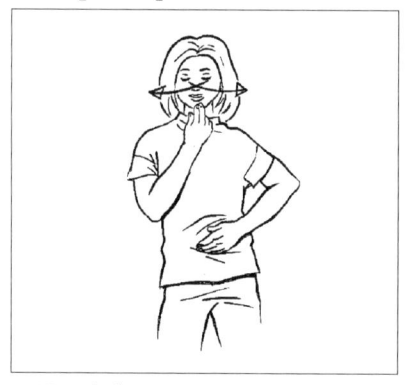

Earth buttons p. 87

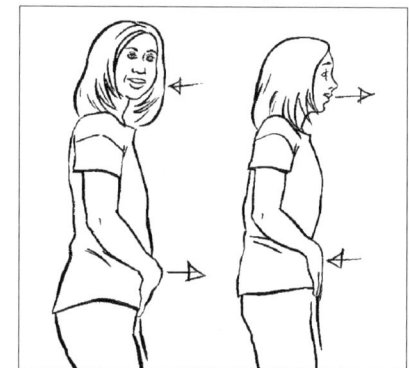

Space buttons p. 95

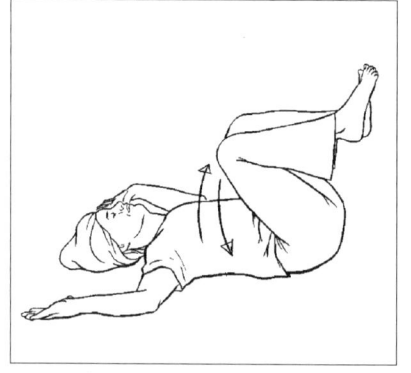

Belly breathing p. 83

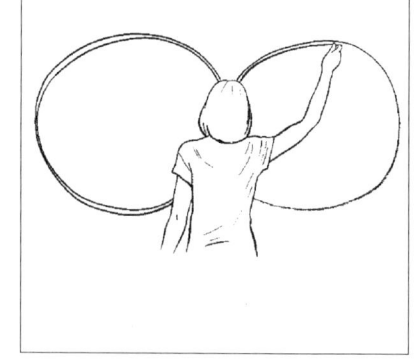

Rocker p. 95

Lazy-8 p. 92

Posttest

✔Read a paragraph. How much can you remember of what you have read?

✔Read another piece aloud and listen to your voice. What does it sound like?

✔Recall a difficult word you have read before. Look up. Can you see the word clearly in your mind's eye?

✔How does it sound and feel now when you read? Do you remember what the words look like?

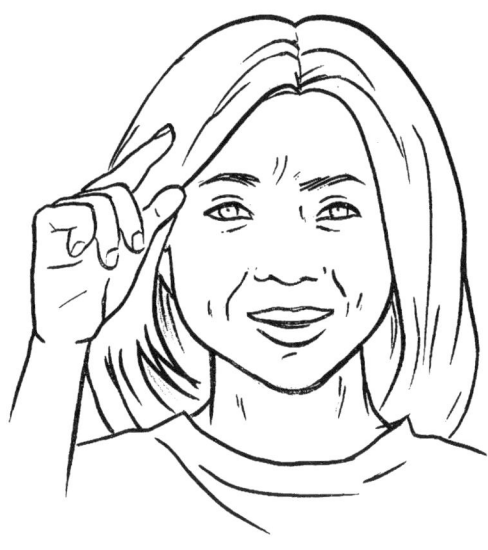

Brain Gym® for better memory

These days our senses are literally bombarded by screaming posters, alarms, TV, crowds of people around us and masses of things to choose from. To protect you against overload, your brain sifts through the information so that you are only aware of the most important information. If your senses are overloaded over a long period, they shut down and no longer remember well.

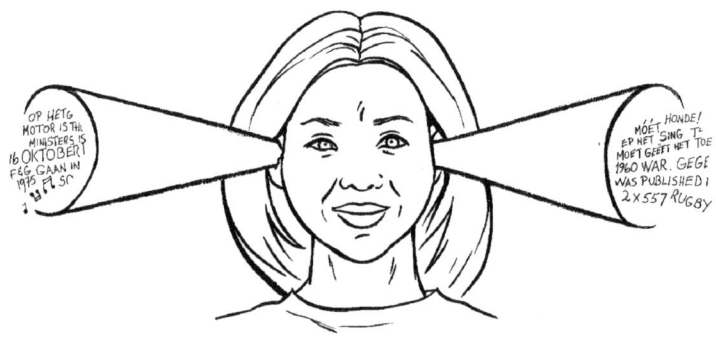

Memory is the end result of good-quality sensory perception. The more of your senses that are observing an event at any one time, the greater the chance that it will make an impression on you and be stored in your memory.

Some people remember names and shopping lists simply by **hearing** them; others remember better if they have first read or **seen** it and still others remember better if they have had emotions or **feelings** about it. These three ways of learning and remembering are also called **auditory**, **visual** and **kinesthetic** perception.

Irrespective of your preferred perception method, if you stimulate all your senses, you avoid overloading and tiring the preferred sense of perception and improve your quality of perception, and with it your memory.

High quality information + emotion = memory

58

Pretest

Observe your surroundings, where you are sitting and reading. Close your eyes and recall, or write down, your impressions without looking again.
✔What did you see?
✔What did you hear?
✔What did you feel – perhaps the wind against your cheek or the chair covering?
✔Of which smells or tastes were you aware?

Brain Gym®

Do these Brain Gym® exercises **slowly** and regularly.

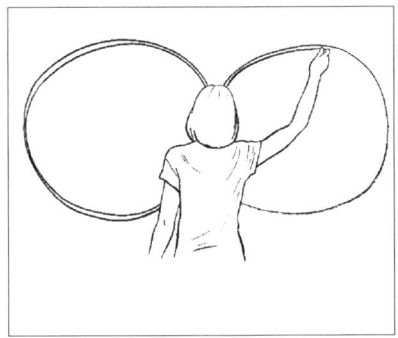

Lazy-8 p. 92

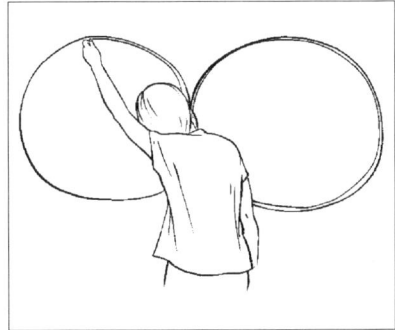

Elephant p. 88

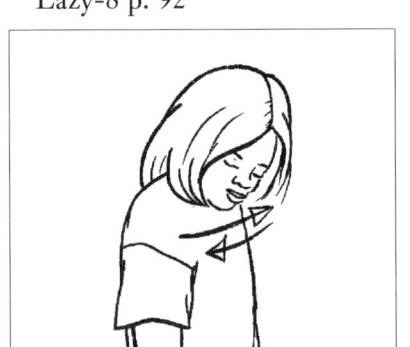

Neck roll p. 93

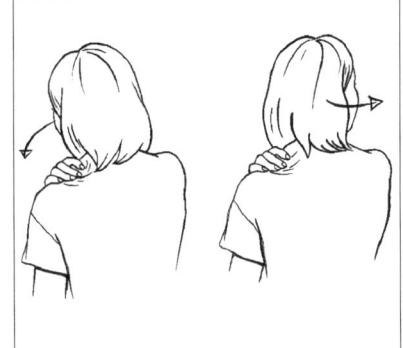

Owl p. 94

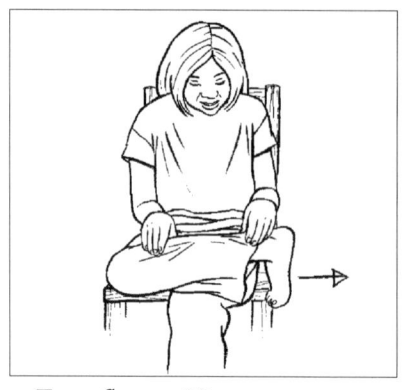

Foot flex p. 89

Grounder p. 90

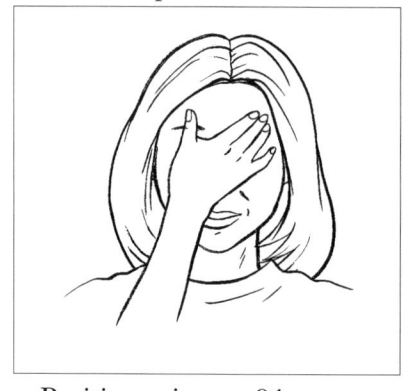

Positive points p. 94

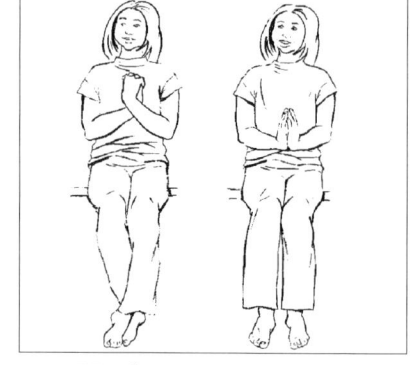

Hook-up p. 91

Posttest

Observe your surroundings, where you are sitting and reading. Close your eyes and recall, or write down, your impressions without looking again.
✔What did you see?
✔What did you hear?
✔What did you feel?
✔Of which smells or tastes were you aware?

Are you now perhaps aware of more things?

Brain Gym® for clear communication

Language is the key to human interaction and a social life, a means to express yourself and to organise your thoughts. Language and thinking develop together, even though language develops a little faster.

The ability to speak is the result of a long, complex process in the brain that takes place over many years. The urge to speak is already clear early on, in babies. If a baby wants to be picked up, or she is wet or hungry, she has to make a plan: she must either get the bottle herself by crawling towards it, or communicate her need to someone who can do something about it.

The start of communication!

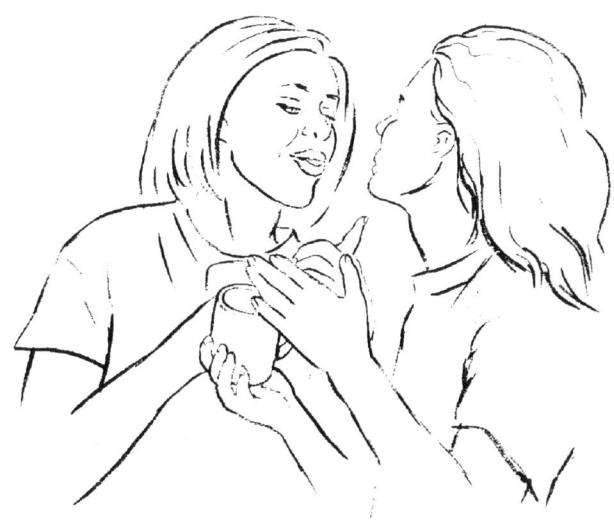

Communication is the ability to express your thoughts so clearly that you (the sender) and the other person (the receiver) attach the same meaning to your words; and to listen in such a way that you (now the receiver) can understand the other person's (now the sender) message the way it was meant.

The left brain is commonly seen as the language brain and the right brain as the interpreting brain. Both are needed to communicate easily and clearly. The left brain focuses on the **parts** of language such as letters, words and names of objects, while the right brain focuses more on the **meaning and possible applications** of language. You also need your back and front brains for good communication – the back brain so that you can observe information through your senses and associate this information with previous experiences and information; and your front brain to use this information by speaking about it, reacting to it, or taking action. When the perceived information is important to you, your lower brain works with all the other parts of your brain so that you can remember it and it can be stored in your memory for future use.

To convert this complex process of perceiving, processing and reacting successfully into words, requires complex neural networks and a relaxed attitude. When you are tense, your survival reflex is activated which means that, among other things, your calf muscles contract and shorten to enable you to fight or flee. Action is then more important than words. Constant stress over a long period can thus restrict your ability to use language and express yourself.

Because the communication process is so complex, there are many sensory network groups that can be tested: your perception networks, your processing networks and your language and reaction networks.

Pretest

✔Look up, down, left and right. How comfortable are your eye movements?

✔Turn your head to the left and listen to the sounds around you.

✔Turn your head to the right and listen again. Do both ears hear equally well?

✔Think of your goal and write a few sentences about it. Is it easy to organise your thoughts and put them into words?

✔In your imagination, tell someone what you want to achieve. Easy or difficult?

Brain Gym®

Do these Brain Gym® exercises **slowly** and regularly.

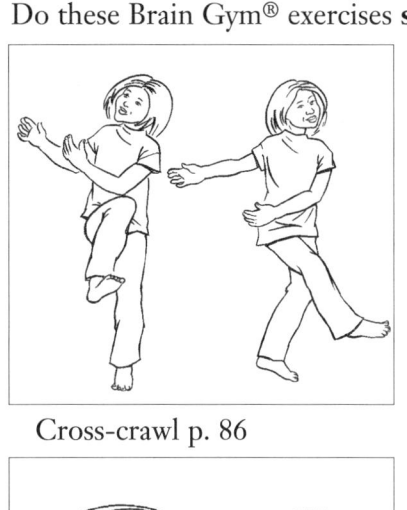

Cross-crawl p. 86

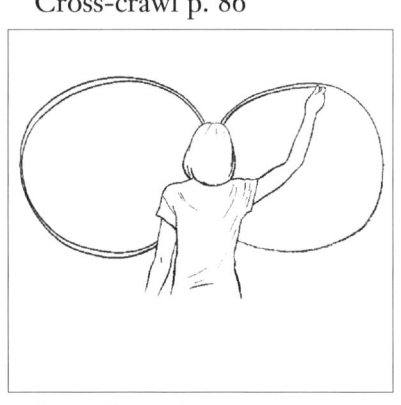

Lazy-8 p. 92

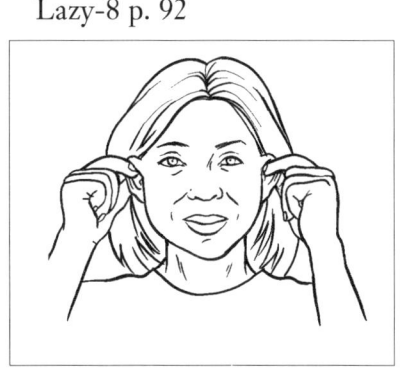

Thinking caps p. 96

Neck roll p. 93

Alphabet-8, p. 80

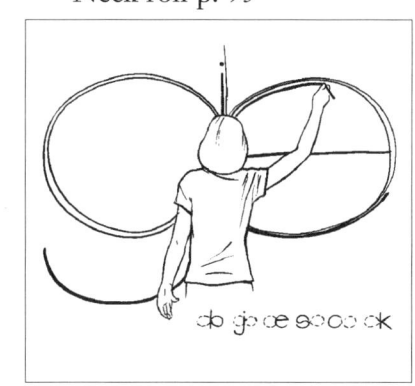

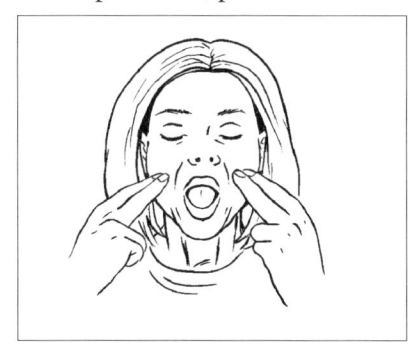

Energy yawn p. 89

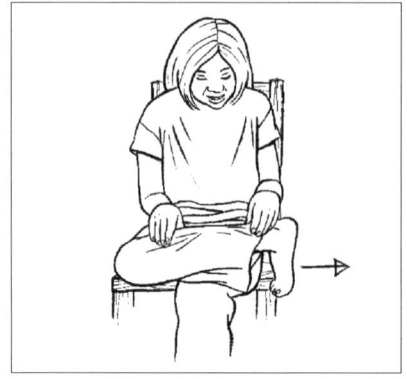 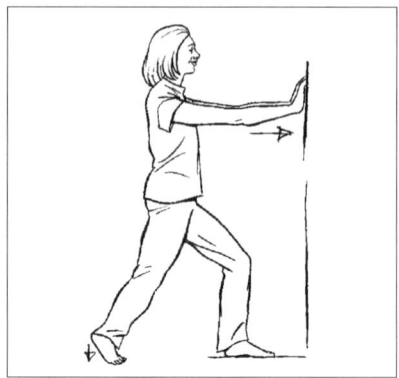

Foot flex p. 89   Calf pump p. 85

Posttest

✔ Look up, down, left and right. How comfortable are your eye movements?

✔ Turn your head to the left and listen to the sounds around you.

✔ Turn your head to the right and listen again. Do both ears hear equally well?

✔ Think of your goal and write a few sentences about it. Is it easy to organise your thoughts and put them into words?

✔ In your imagination, tell someone what you want to achieve. Easy or difficult?

Brain Gym® for organisation

Organisation is the ability to pay attention to numerous tasks and complete them within a given period. Some of the most important components of the ability to organise are determining **what** to do, by **when** it should be done, in which **order** tasks should be tackled, **who** must do what and exactly **how** they must be done; to ensure that the end product is satisfactory and up to standard.

This gift to be able to weave several threads into a coherent whole presupposes good cooperation between your upper and lower brain, as well as your upper and lower body. When your upper and lower body do not work well together, your balance is disturbed and you feel distracted and fragmented. You bump into furniture and doors, you pick up and drop tasks, you feel unsure of yourself, battle to organise your surroundings, and for these reasons soon feel overwhelmed.

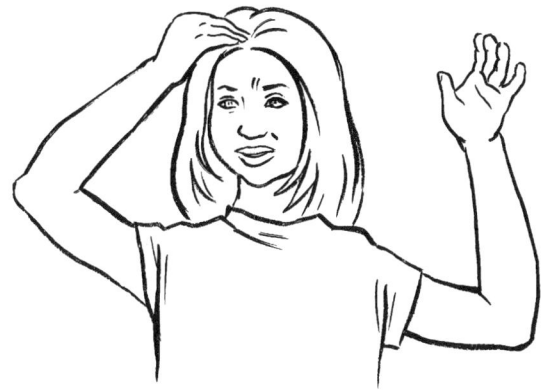

The following Brain Gym® exercises strengthen the nerve pathways between your upper and lower brain and all your senses, which in turn strengthen your balance and sense of direction, so that you feel centred and in control of yourself. When you have control over your position in space, you are organised internally and it is therefore much easier to organise your surroundings.

Pretest

✔Think about your goal and walk while you do so. Be aware of how you are walking: is your weight on your whole foot, or more to the heel or the outside of your foot?

✔Are you walking purposefully or dragging yourself along?

✔Think about all the things that have to happen before you can reach your goal and decide where to begin. Do you know where to start, or is it all darkness?

Brain Gym®

Do the following Brain Gym® exercises **slowly** and regularly.

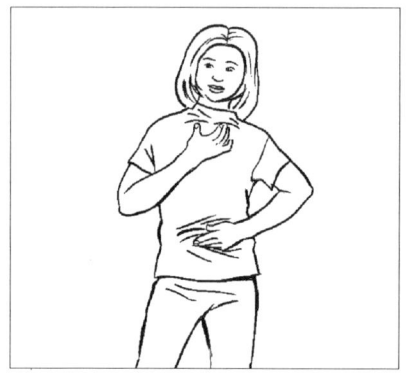

Brain buttons p. 84

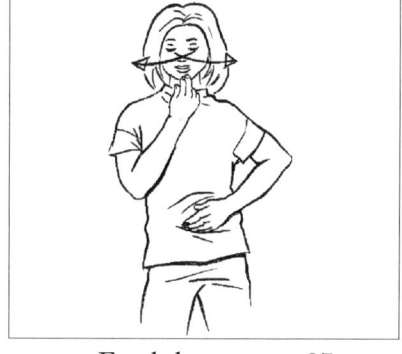

Earth buttons p. 87

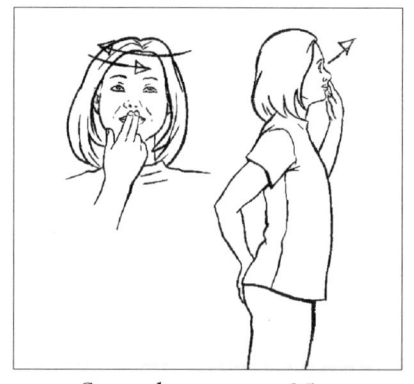

Space buttons p. 95

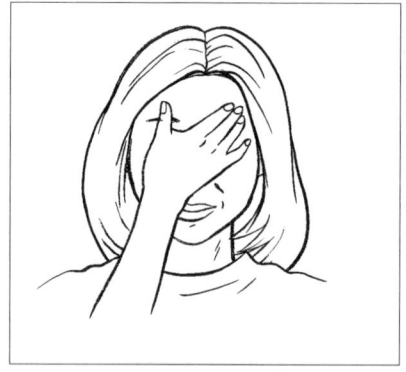

Positive points p. 94

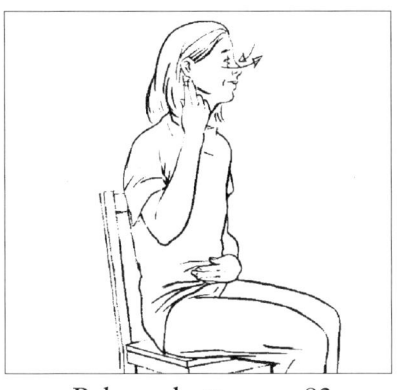

Balance buttons p. 82

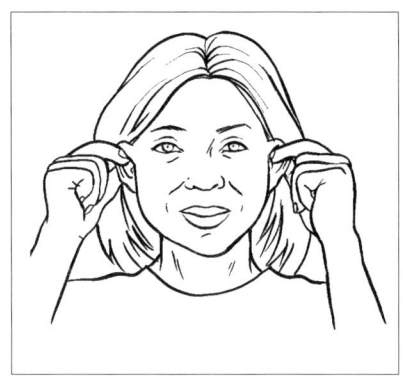

Thinking caps p. 96

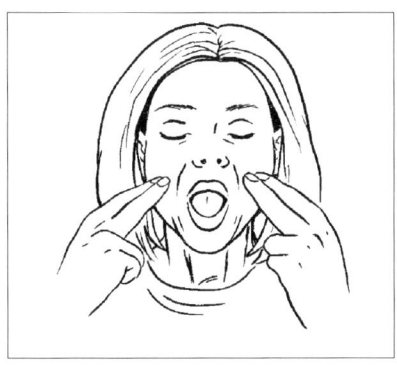

Energy yawn p. 89

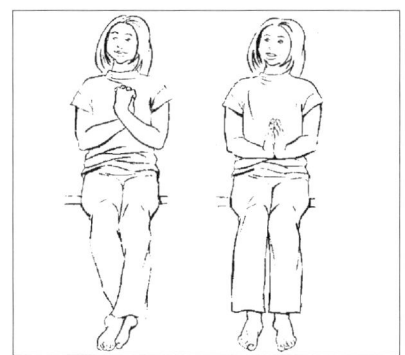

Hook-up p. 91

Posttest

✔Think about your goal and walk while you do so. Be aware of how you are walking: is your weight on your whole foot, or more to the heel or outside of your foot?

✔Are you walking purposefully or dragging yourself along?

✔Think about all the things that have to happen before you can reach your goal and decide where to begin. Where must you start?

Brain Gym® for better concentration

How is it that some people can anticipate and avoid problems and, at the same time, be aware of opportunities and grab them enthusiastically, while so many others seem to stumble from crisis to crisis? It is almost as if the first group runs on high-octane fuel and is always at the right place, at the right time.

These lucky people have effective integration between their back and front brains, and a good flow of cerebrospinal fluid. Cerebrospinal fluid carries hormones and nutrients to the brain, cools the brain and removes waste products, enabling these fortunate souls to function optimally. The movement of cerebrospinal fluid is influenced by such factors as body movement, the contraction and relaxation of calf muscles and the quality of breathing.

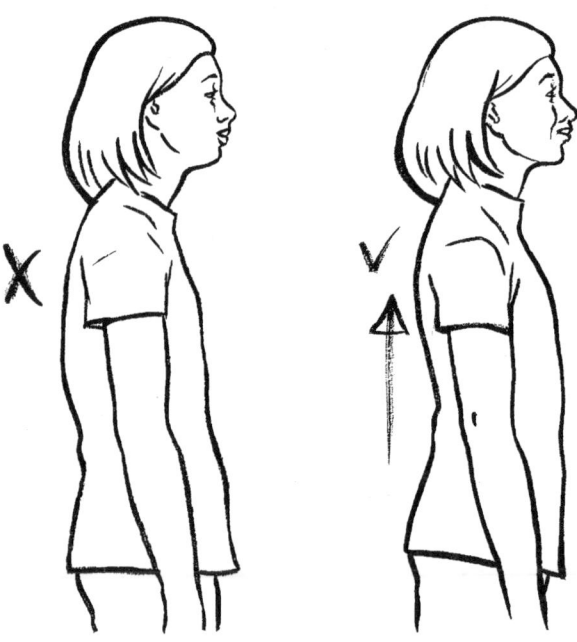

The back brain (like the right brain) is more instinctive and intuitive and stores raw, unprocessed data all at the same time for later processing. The front brain (like the left brain) is more selective and processes experiences rationally by analysing them logically and verbalising them. It is only when the back and front brains work easily with the senses and other parts of the brain, that you can concentrate with more focus.

A person's carriage and posture often reveal a lack of back- and front-brain integration.

Children who tend to be easily distracted are often right- and back-brain dominant, which means that they observe *everything* around them and cannot distinguish between what is **important now** and what is not. They just try harder and harder with less and less results, because their natural wiring prevents **selective** observation. In addition, they usually process new data by **moving** – rocking, running around and uncontrolled body movements. The result: a "hyperactive child with attention deficit disorder".

The following group of Brain Gym® movements have been proved effective, worldwide, in strengthening nerve networks to improve concentration and completion of tasks.

Pretest

✔If you stand up straight in your usual manner, can you draw a straight line from your ear through your shoulder, hip and ankle, or is it a zigzag line?

✔Choose an object close to you and focus on it. Do your thoughts wander or do they stay focused?

✔Continue focusing on the object, but be aware of other objects and sounds in the vicinity. Can you handle wide-angle focusing without losing awareness of the original object, or do you lose your focus when you extend your observation field?

✔If you start doing one task, do you complete it before starting with the next, or do you jump from task to task without completing any?

69

Brain Gym®

Do the following Brain Gym® exercises daily, and **slowly**, for at least 2 months.

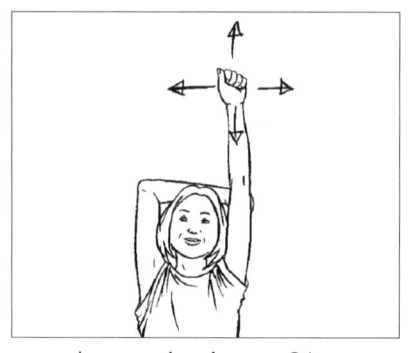

Arm activation p. 81

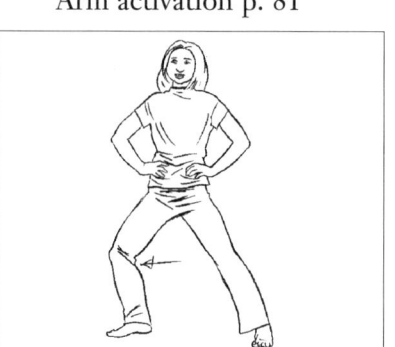

Grounder p. 90

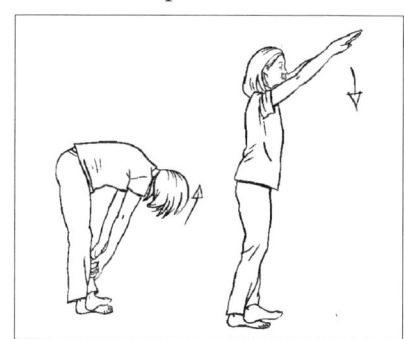

Owl p. 94

Gravity glider p. 90

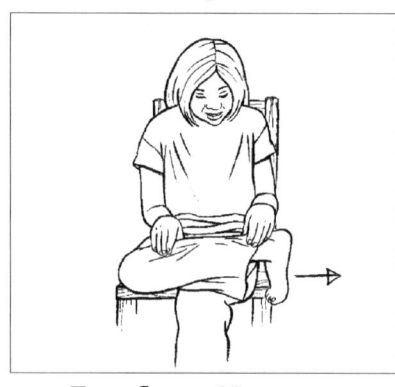

Foot flex p. 89

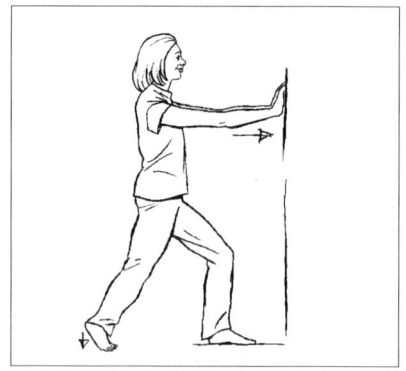

Calf pump p. 85

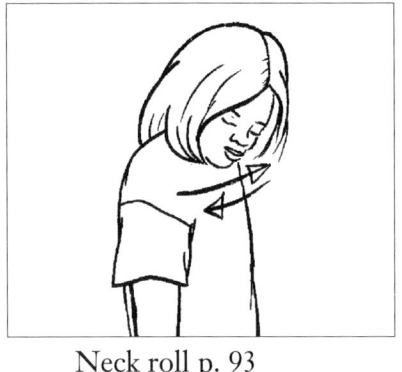
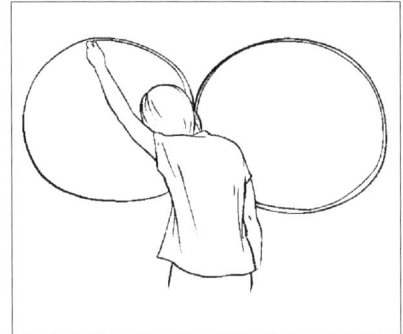

Neck roll p. 93   Elephant p. 88

Posttest

✔ If you stand up straight in your usual manner, can you draw a straight line from your ear through your shoulder, hip and ankle, or is it still a zigzag line?

✔ Choose an object close to you and focus on it, but also be aware of other objects and sounds in the vicinity. Can you handle wide-angle focusing and still be aware of the original object?

Brain Gym® for banishing depression

Depression is described in the dictionary as a **process** of decline and repression, characterised by low energy levels, reduced initiative, feelings of inadequacy and a restricted outlook.

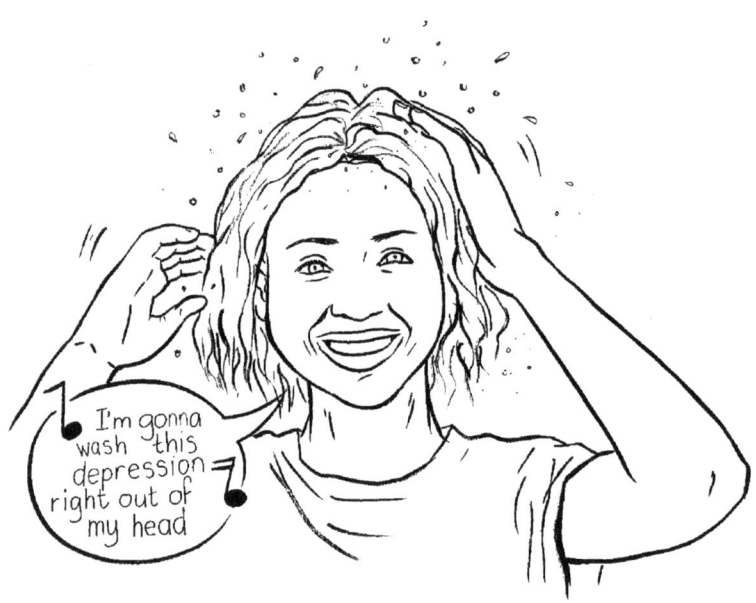

The causes of depression are numerous and can range from the death of a loved one, moving house, unemployment, abuse and rejection to the wrong choice of occupation or marital partner or the absence of a partner. In "Brain Gym® for banishing depression" the focus is on those things that are common to everyone who has ever experienced depression. This includes physical symptoms such as a hunched posture, downcast eyes, tiredness, passivity and the "big thirst", as well as psychological symptoms such as negativity and hopelessness.

To feel depressed can be a great gift if you start searching for the **source** or **original file** of this feeling. Often the source is the result of an inner battle between what you want to be or know you can be and your current situation. The difference between what **is** and what **can be**, leads to an inner knowledge that a part of your being is repressed and that you are capable of much more than is at present being realised in your life.

You can spend years in therapy, digging to find the root of your underachievement and feelings of depression. Unfortunately you cannot change your past, but with the right guidance you can change the intensity of the effects your past has on your life. What about the here and now while you are engaged in self-examination? This is where *Brain Gym® for all* can make a meaningful contribution to your life: it offers the **possibility** of feeling different – with the creation of new files.

You can do it!
Start today.

Pretest

✔How do you feel now? Write down one or more words.
✔Look around you. Are the curtains open and is there enough fresh air and light in the room?
✔How do you usually sit or stand – upright with your head held high, or do you look down?
✔How much water did you drink yesterday: 6-8 glasses?
✔When last did you do something new, such as rearranging your furniture, having meals and tea breaks at different times, taking another route to the shops, or simply walking in the garden and smelling a flower?

Brain Gym®

Do the following Brain Gym® movements (10 minutes daily, for at least 6 weeks) to alter your posture and eye movements, to integrate your entire brain and in so doing create fresh new networks so that you can realise your true being and take on the rest of your life with zest!

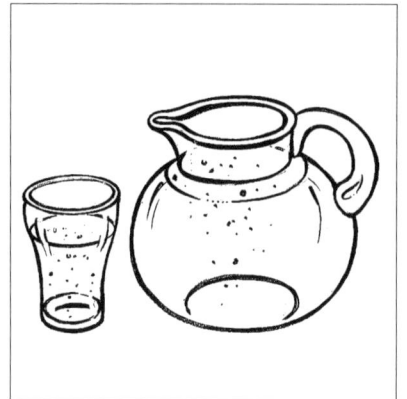

Drink water

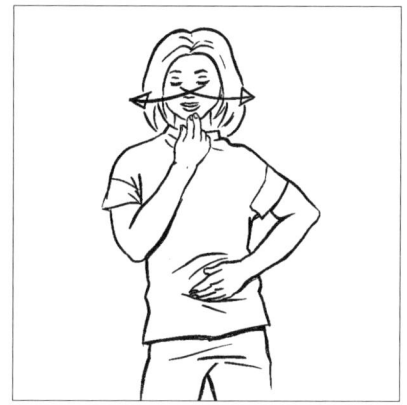

Brain buttons p. 84

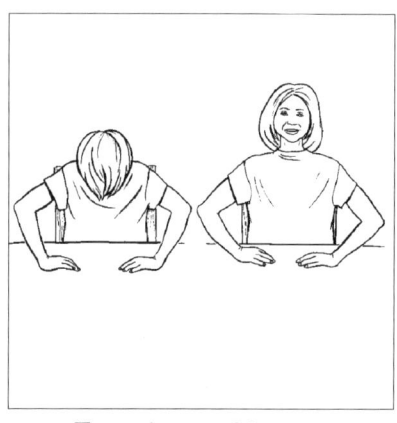

Energiser p. 88

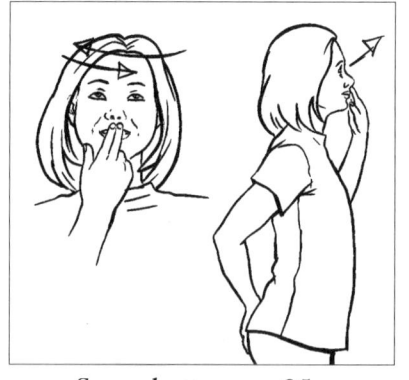

Earth buttons p. 87

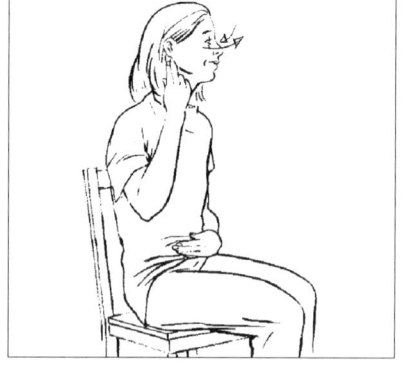

Space buttons p. 95

Balance buttons p. 82

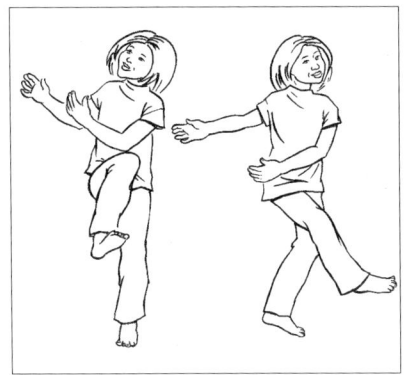

Cross-crawl p. 86

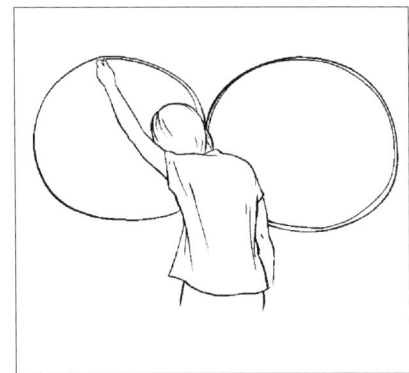

Elephant p. 88

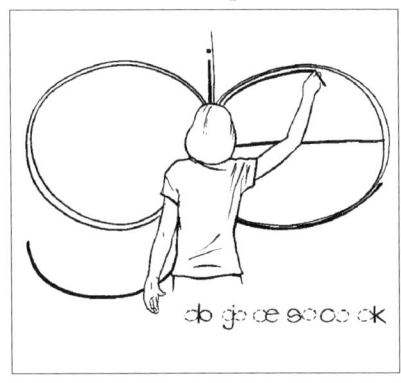

Alphabet-8 p. 80

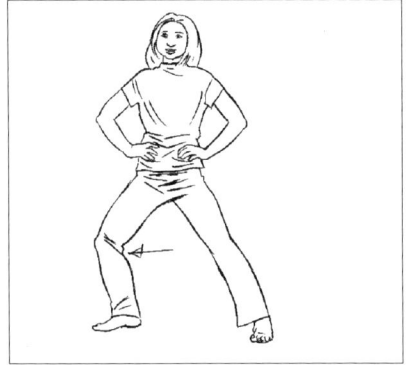

Grounder p. 90

Posttest

✔Look around you. Are the curtains open and is there enough fresh air and light in the room?

✔How do you sit or stand now – straighter, with your head held high?

✔To do the Brain Gym® exercises is something new. How do you feel now, compared to the pretest?

Continue to drink a little more water, spend more time in nature, and do your exercises every day.

Brain Gym® for eliminating stress and anxiety

Fear is the little darkroom where negatives are developed
M. Pritchard

When you think about the future, it can be with anticipation or with horror. The way you think about it, depends on **what** you think about and **what** you wonder about.

If you can think of your life as a film and of yourself as the director creating it, is it not up to you whether it is a thriller or an adventure? The director has an idea he expands on and colours in to make a masterpiece, but this masterpiece started with a basic idea. This basic idea is your deepest convictions. And these **convictions or knowledge** drive you to carry on every day and they are also what you use as criteria when making decisions.

When your basic conviction is that "the world conspires to make my life a party", you will approach life with that attitude. But when your basic conviction is: "life and everybody in it are out to get me/hurt me", then that is the standpoint from which you go forward to meet your future. If you are the director and the script says: "everybody and everything is against me", it evokes intense fear and tension, because "it is only a matter of time before the worst happens". The question is not, therefore, **if** it will happen, but **when** it will happen.

The underlying emotion fuelling such a conviction is **fear**. Fear, in turn, creates worry and worry induces stress and anxiety. On the other hand, when a person believes that the world and all people (or at least most of them) in it are well disposed towards him, he is fuelled by **joy**.

Someone who (mainly unconsciously) believes the world to be an unkind place, is motivated by fear and can, as the quote says, develop a negative film in his darkroom. This is what happens in reality: your future is like a blank videotape – what you think about creates the possibility that it can happen. Whether you are driven by fear or joy, your future is still just a possibility. Your thoughts, your convictions and what you believe **together** make your life an adventure or a thriller.

You might say: "But what if . . . because it has happened before." But what about: "What if it doesn't . . . even if it has happened before"?

Who knows?

Anxiety and stress (like a feeling of depression) usually have very deep roots. It may sometimes be difficult to fight it by yourself, in which case professional help is recommended. But because you know that, using Brain Gym®, you can delete and edit wiring and files, you could perhaps, with the help of *Brain Gym® for all*, start to consider the possibility that you (the director of any age) can start your new script with a brand-new conviction and knowledge of:

What if . . . because then it can . . .

Pretest

Martin Luther King changed not only his own life, but also those of many other people with his words: "I have a dream . . ."

✔What is your dream? What do you dream about in terms of your:
✔ relationships
✔ social life
✔ work and occupation
✔ health
✔ spiritual life
✔Can you consider the possibility of change and a different future?
✔On a scale of 0–10, how relaxed and peaceful do you feel at the moment?
0 = very stressed and 10 = relaxed and peaceful.

Brain Gym®

Do the Brain Gym® exercises **slowly**, every day, for at least 2 months.

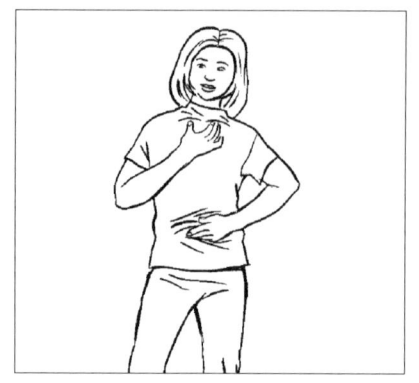

Brain buttons p. 84

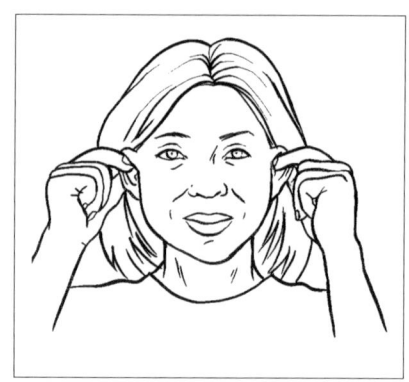

Thinking caps p. 96

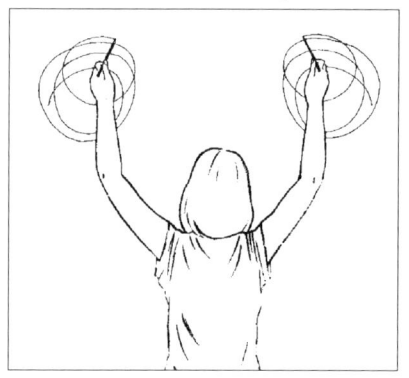

Double doodle p. 86

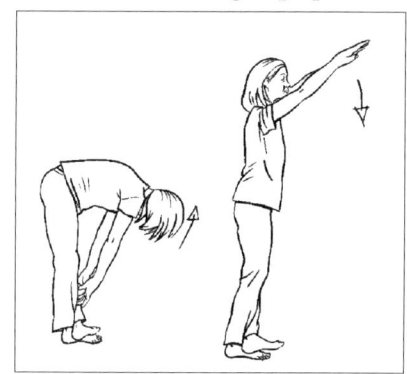

Gravity glider p. 90

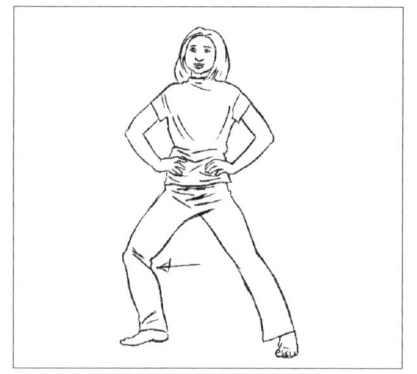

Grounder p. 90

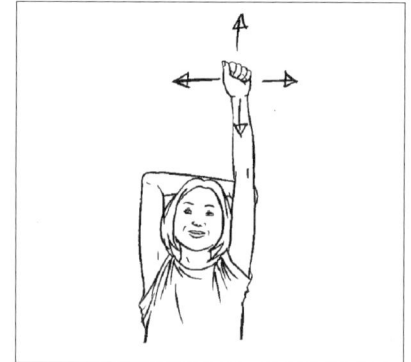

Arm activation p. 81

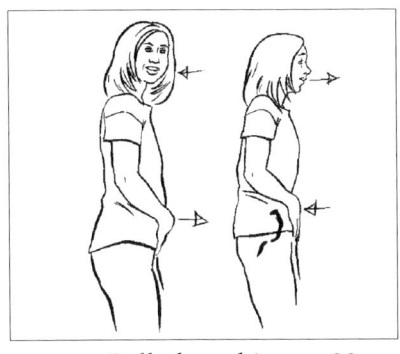

Belly breathing p. 83

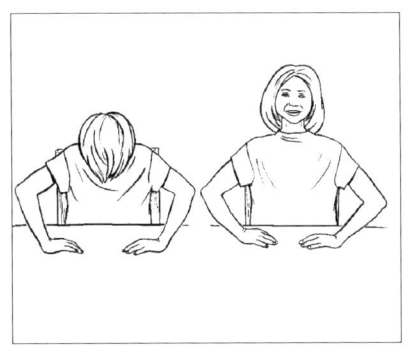

Energiser p. 88

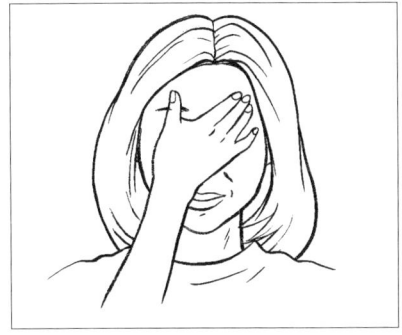

Thinking caps p. 96

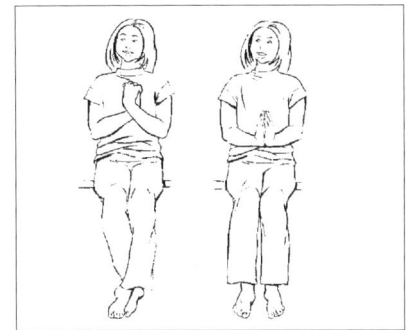

Hook-up p. 91

Posttest

✔How do you feel and think now?
✔Measure your level of relaxation again on a scale of 0–10. The number changed, didn't it?

A wise person once said:
Reason is the greatest gift of all –
With reason comes understanding.
With understanding comes caring.
With caring comes love.
Go forth in love.

Brain Gym®

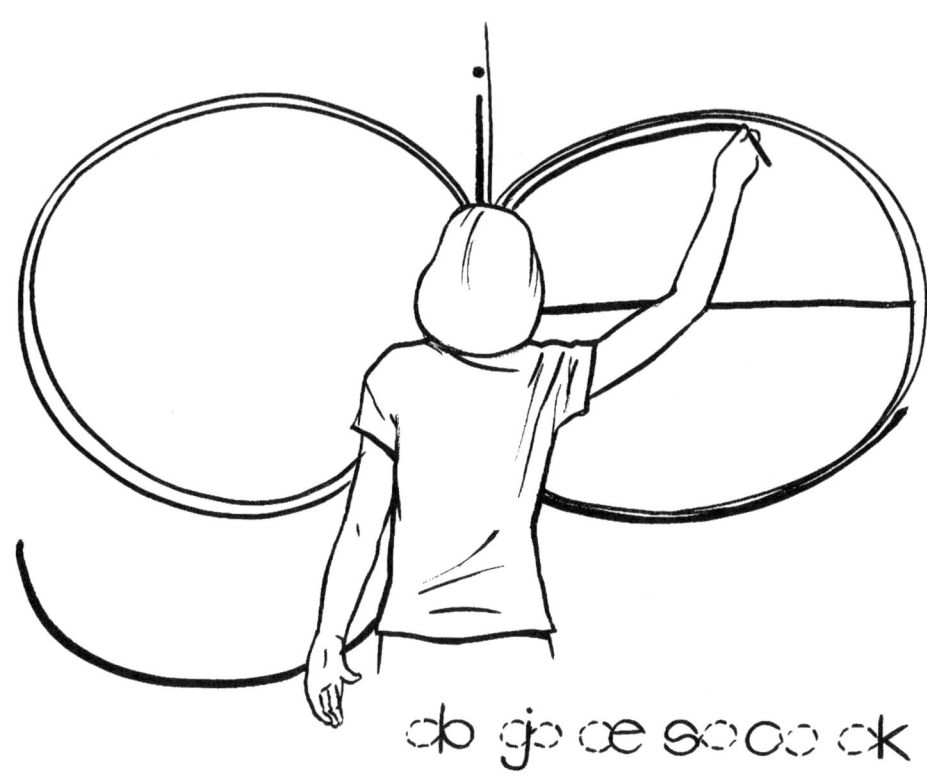

Alphabet-8

Do a few Lazy-8s (see p. 92) – first with one hand, then with the other. Start in the centre of the Lazy-8 and form the letters of the alphabet over one another on the curves of the circles. Make a Lazy-8 between each completed letter to improve fluency of writing and relaxation.

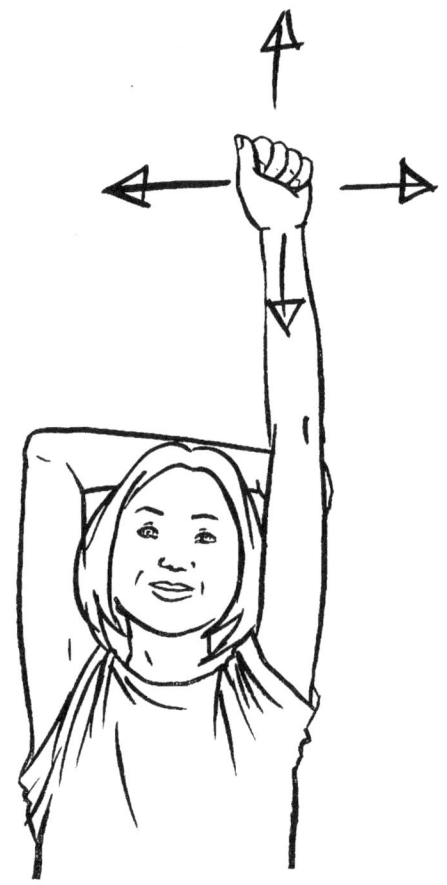

Arm activation

Hold one arm straight up next to your ear and place the other as shown in the picture. Your arms work against one another, in opposite directions, so that your arm, shoulder and back muscles lengthen. Press first one and then the other arm forwards, backwards, left and right for at least 8 seconds each time while exhaling.

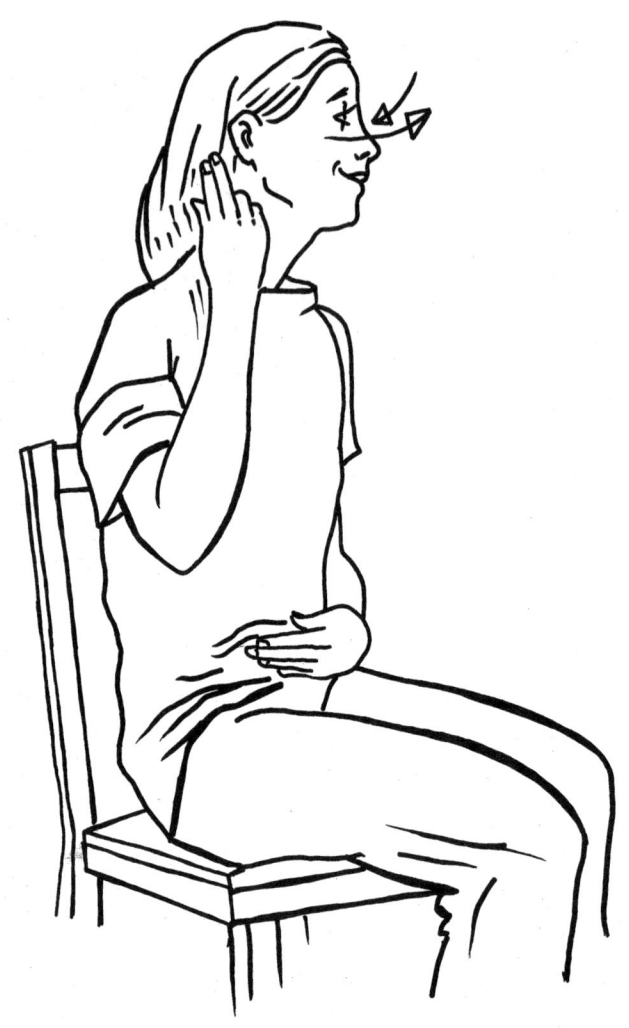

Balance buttons

Place one hand on your navel and the other on the soft hollow where the skull and the neck meet just behind your ear. Keeping your head upright, move your eyes horizontally from left to right while softly stimulating the hollow. Change hands and stimulate the balance button on the other side as well.

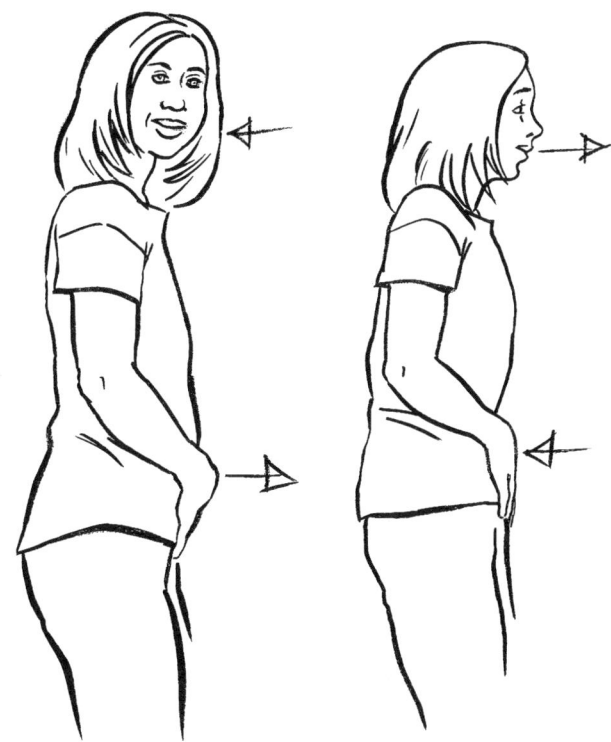

Belly breathing

Place your hands on your stomach. Think of your stomach as a bal-
loon you are blowing up when you breathe in and deflate when you
breathe out. As you inhale, your hands will be pushed forwards and
as you exhale they will fall back slightly.

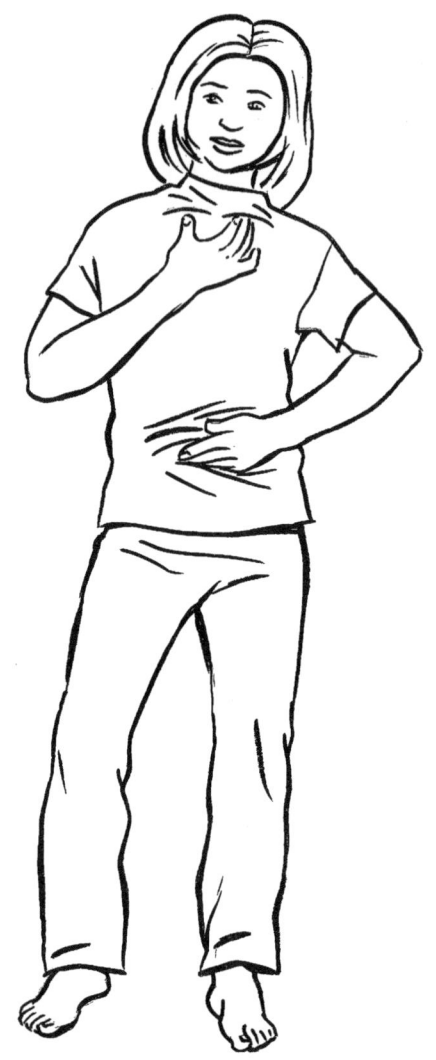

Brain buttons

Place one hand on your navel (this stimulates balance) and, using the thumb and index finger of your other hand, stimulate the two hollows just under your collarbone, on either side of your breastbone.

Calf pump

Stand up straight with your hands against a wall at shoulder height. Stretch one leg to the back and lift your heel. Bend the knee of the front leg. Press firmly against the wall with your hands while you press your heel flat against the floor for 8 seconds. Lift your back heel and straighten your front knee as you breathe in. Breathe out, bending your front knee again and pressing your back heel to the ground. Repeat for the other side.

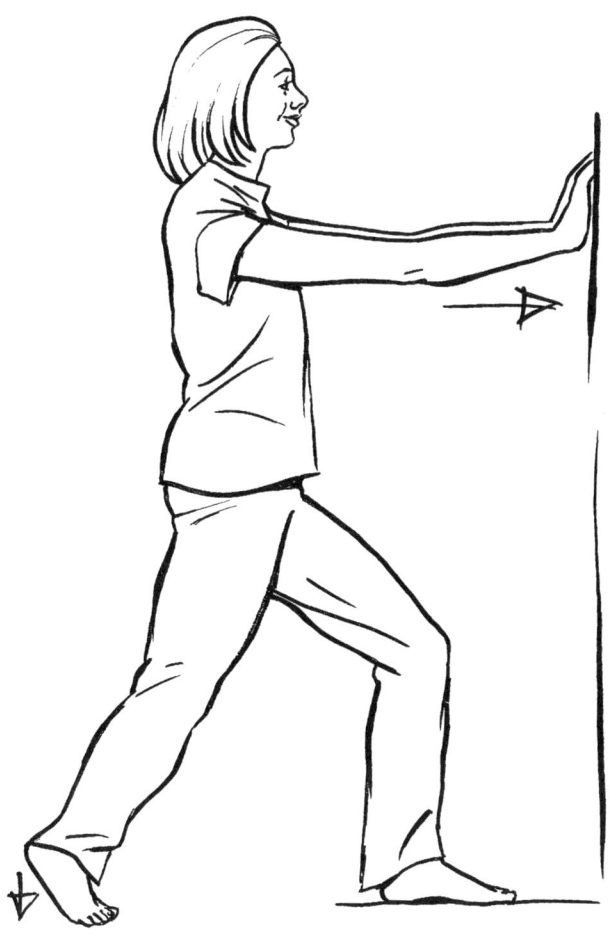

Cross-crawl

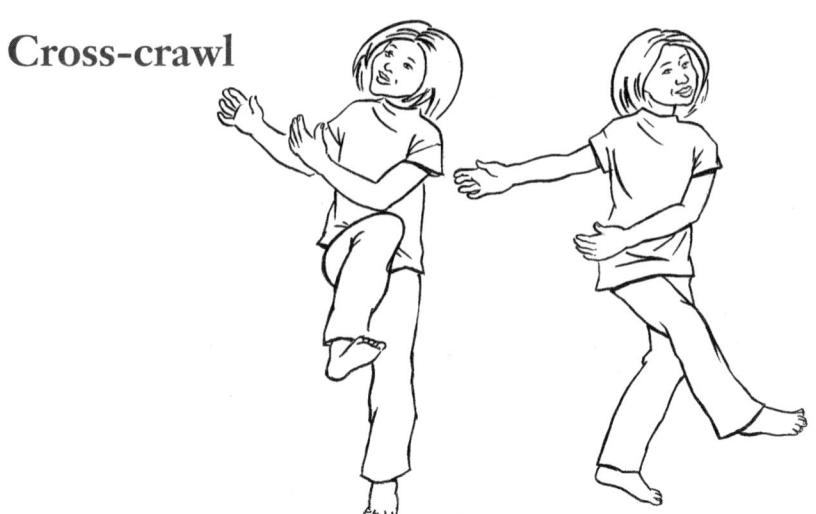

Sit or stand up straight. Touch your right knee with your left elbow, then your left knee with your right elbow. Continue to cross your body midline slowly.

Double doodle

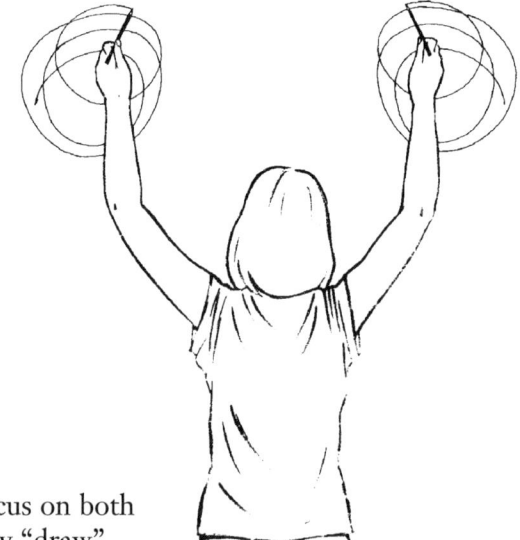

Keeping your head still, focus on both hands as you simultaneously "draw" large circles that are mirror images of each other. When your hands work easily together, but in opposite directions, you will make large, free-form, symmetrical doodle patterns.

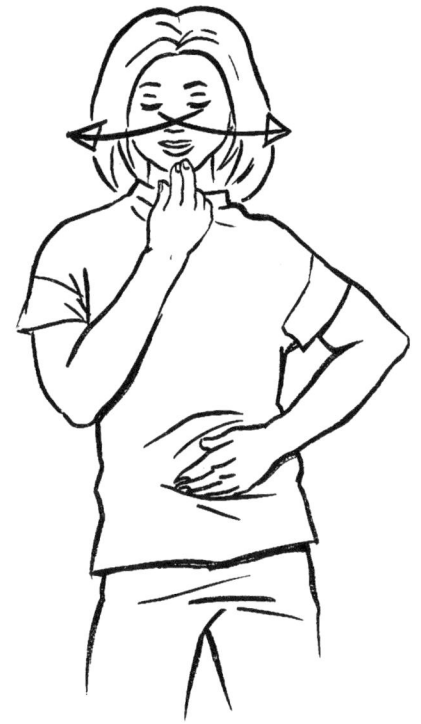

Earth buttons

Place one hand on your navel and place your other hand on your chin. Looking down, move your eyes slowly from left to right a few times.

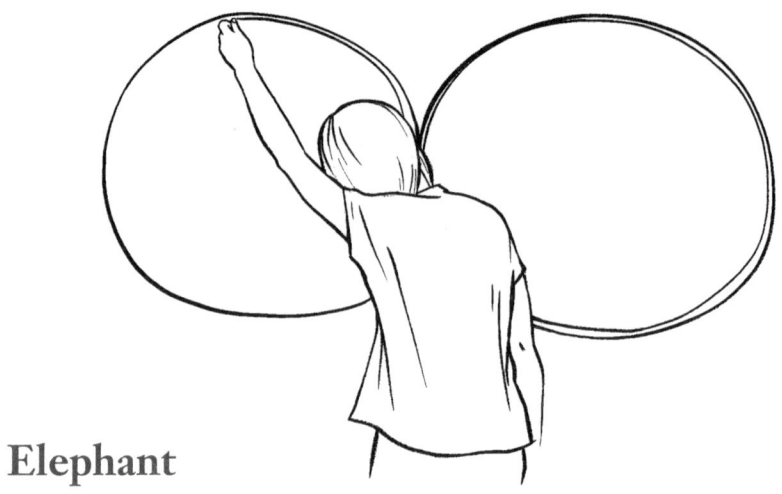

Elephant

Sit or stand up straight, with one arm stretched out and pressed to your ear, eyes focusing on the tips of your fingers and beyond. As for Lazy-8 (see p. 92), moving from your midline, make large circular movements to left and right, always moving upwards at the centre, where the two circles touch. Change arms and repeat the movement.

Energiser

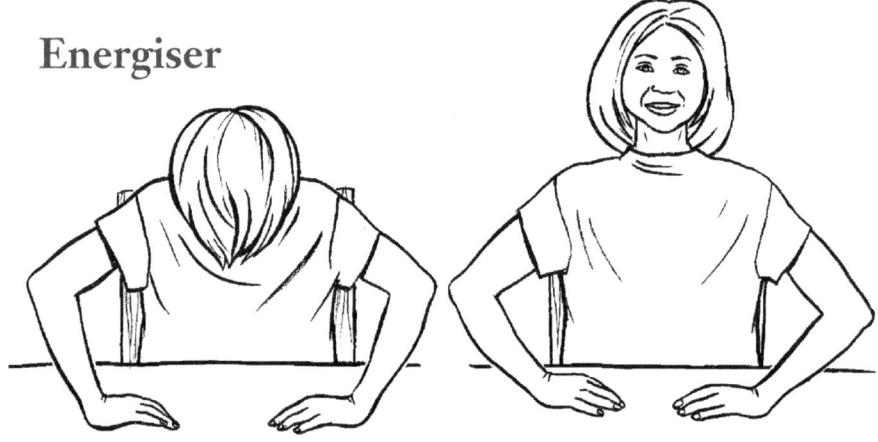

Sit comfortably on a chair, head bent and back hunched, and place your hands (fingertips facing) on the table. Breathe in deeply and slowly as you raise your head and eyes, straightening your back. Breathe out slowly as you lower your head. Relax. Repeat several times.

Energy yawn

Pretend to yawn, close your eyes tightly and massage your jaw-bone, using circular movements around your upper and lower molars. As you massage, give a deep, relaxed yawn.

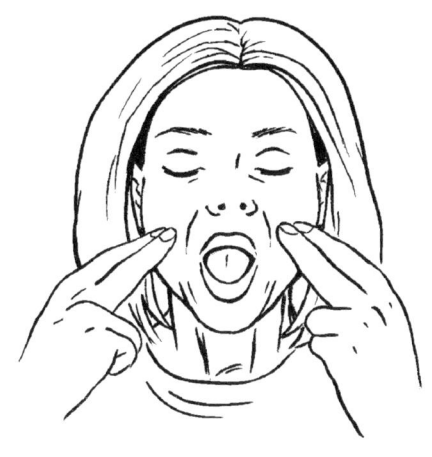

Foot flex

Sit up straight and rest one leg on the other, with your ankle on your knee. Hold your calf muscle between your thumbs and fingers. Massage the muscle, moving one hand towards your knee and the other towards your ankle. Alternately flex and point your foot while massaging.

If you find it difficult to do the foot flex yourself, the movement can be adapted so that somebody else does the massaging. Lie on your stomach on a bed, with your legs stretched out. The helper massages your calf simultaneously with both hands, towards knee and ankle, while you flex and point your foot. Repeat for the other leg.

Gravity glider

Sit or stand with your back bent, ankles crossed and arms relaxed. Inhale slowly, straighten your back and, following your hands with your eyes, lift your arms up in the air. Breathe out slowly as you bend forwards again and relax your arms. Repeat several times.

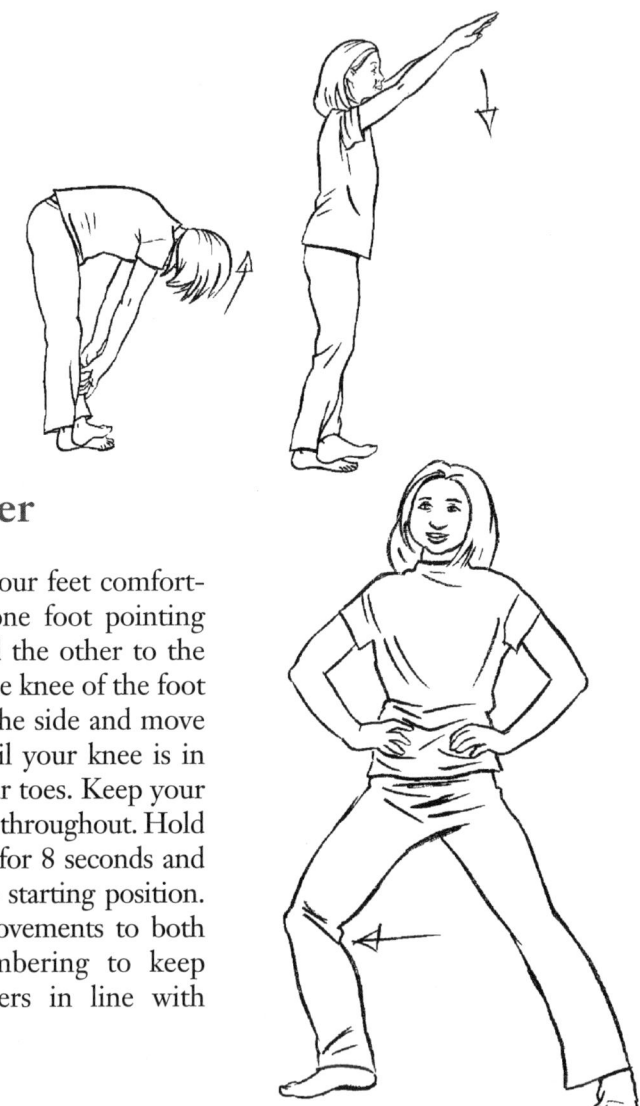

Grounder

Stand with your feet comfortably apart, one foot pointing forwards and the other to the side. Bend the knee of the foot pointing to the side and move sideways until your knee is in line with your toes. Keep your body upright throughout. Hold this position for 8 seconds and return to the starting position. Do a few movements to both sides, remembering to keep your shoulders in line with your hips.

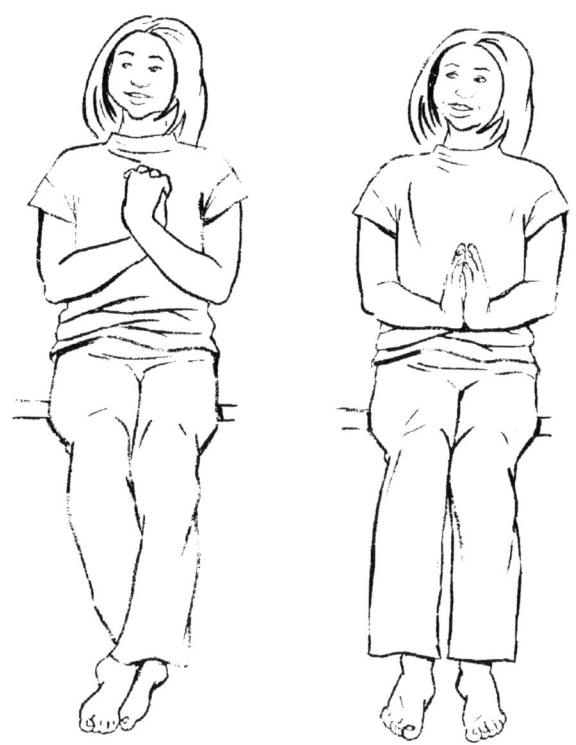

Hook-up

Sit or lie comfortably with your ankles crossed. Stretch your arms out in front of you, the backs of your hands together and your thumbs facing downwards. Turn your hands so that your palms are together and interlace your fingers. Bend your hands down and inwards towards your chest until you are sitting like the figure in the illustration. Relax your shoulders and place your tongue against the highest part of your palate. Breathe slowly and deeply.

After several breaths, uncross your hands and ankles, rest your fingertips against one another and take a last deep breath.

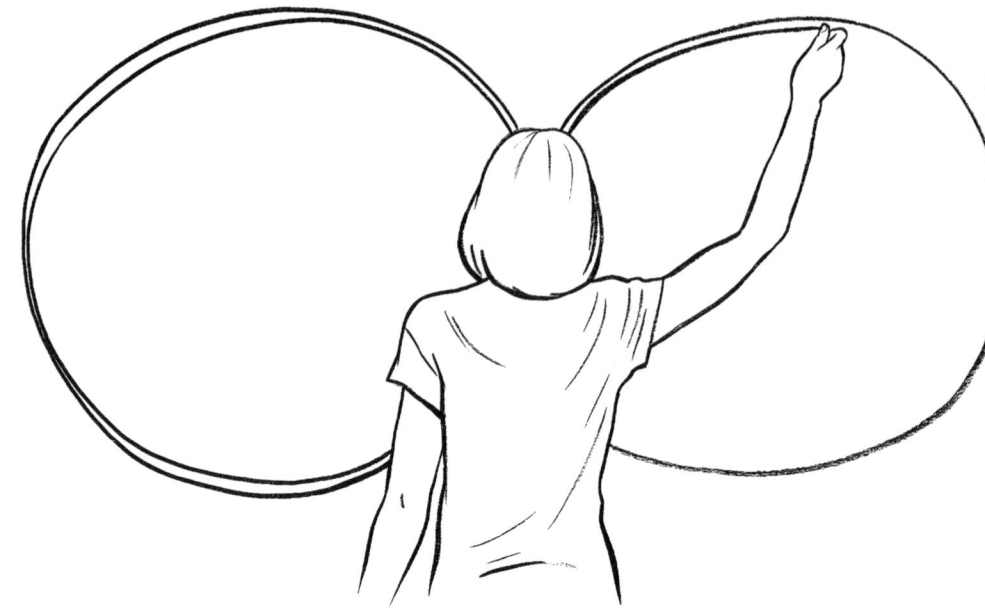

Lazy-8

Stand up straight and hold your thumb out in front of you, at eye level. Look at your thumb as you move it in a large circle around your left eye and then around your right eye. Repeat a few times, with both hands.

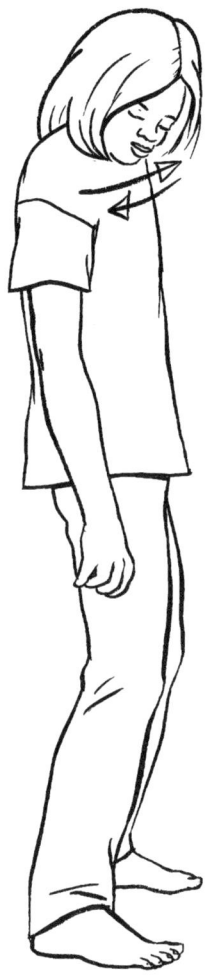

Neck roll

Sit or stand up straight. Imagine that your head is a heavy metal ball and your neck a strong piece of string. Now move your head slowly in a rolling movement to your left shoulder and then to your right shoulder. Lengthen your neck muscles as much as possible and remember to breathe deeply.

Owl

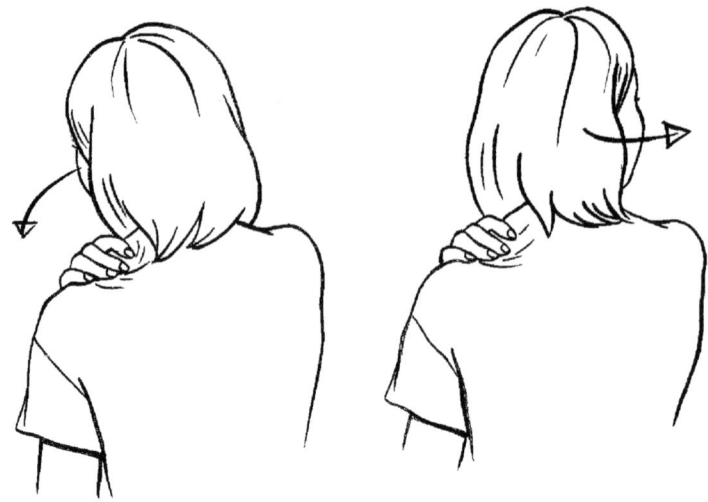

Sit or stand up straight. Massage the large, and often painful, shoulder muscle from your neck to the end of your shoulder. While you massage, keep your head upright and turn it as far as possible to the left, so that you can see over your shoulder. Then slowly turn it back as far as possible to the right to look over your right shoulder as well. Say "Mmmmm . . ." out loud and listen to your voice, turning your head from side to side as you do so. Repeat on the other side.

Positive points

The positive points are halfway between your eyebrows and your hairline, directly in line with the midpoint of your eyes when you look forward. Stimulate these points with both hands or, as shown in the illustration, the thumb and index finger of one hand.

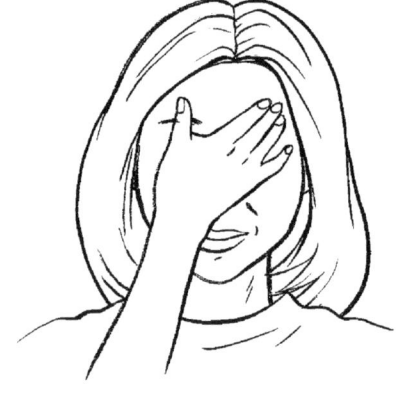

Rocker

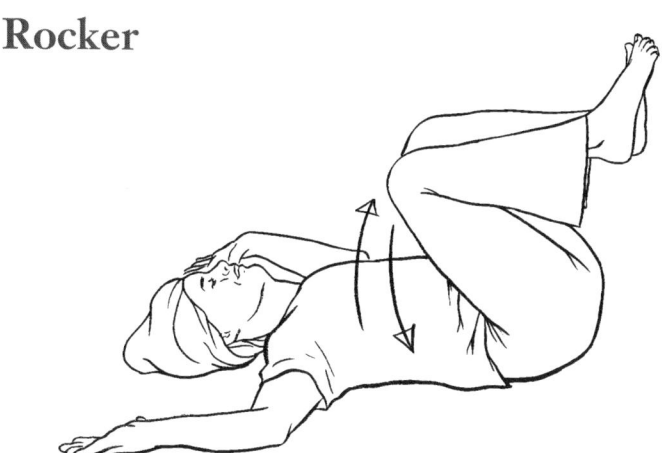

Lie flat on your back on a thick mat or bed and pull your knees up to your chest, as far as you can. Keeping your knees up and your shoulders flat on the bed or mat, swing your hips from one side to the other. Do not stop breathing; breathe normally.

Space buttons

Place one hand on your coccyx (this stimulates the flow of cerebrospinal fluid) and the other between your upper lip and your nose. Look upwards and move your eyes from left to right a few times.

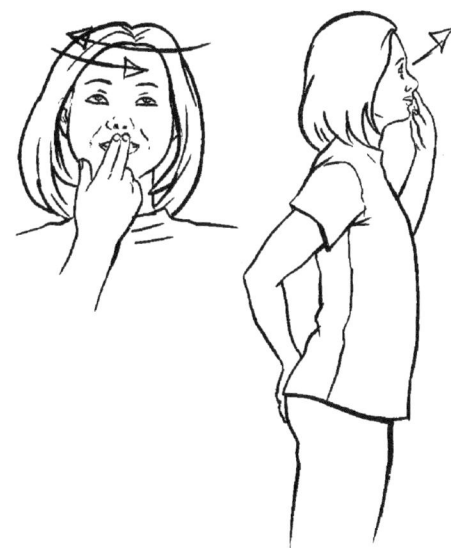

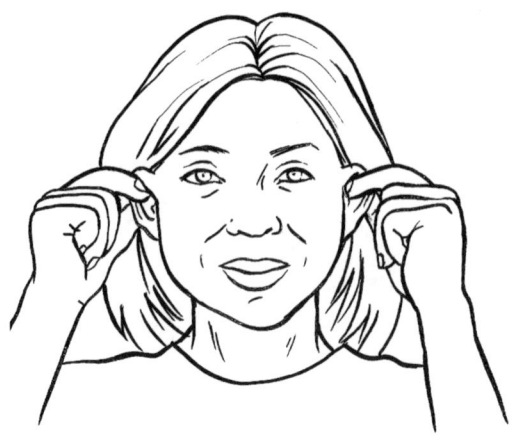

Thinking caps

Sit or stand up straight and hold your ears between your thumbs and index fingers. Massage the entire ear firmly a few times, from top to bottom. Your ears could become red and warm as a result of the increased bloodflow and neural stimulation.

Bibliography

Armstrong, Thomas. *7 Kinds of Smart*. New York: Penguin Books, 1993.

Bandler, Richard and Grinder, John. *Reframing: NLP and the Transformation of Meaning*, Moab, Ut.: Real People Press, 1982.

Buzan, Tony. *Make the Most of Your Mind*. New York: Simon & Schuster, 1988.

De Jager, Melodie. *Mind Dynamics*. Cape Town: Human & Rousseau, 2002

Dennison, Gail E. and Dennison, Paul E. *Brain Gym Handbook*. Ventura, CA: Edu-Kinesthetics, Inc., 1989.

Dennison, Gail E. and Dennison, Paul E. *Brain Gym (Teachers' Edition)*. Ventura, CA: Edu-Kinesthetics, Inc., 1989.

Dennison, Gail E. and Dennison, Paul E. *Switching On*. Ventura, CA: Edu-Kinesthetics, Inc., 1981.

Hannaford, Carla. *Smart Moves*. Arlington, Virginia: Great Ocean Publishers, 1995.

Hannaford, Carla. *The Dominance Factor*. Arlington, Virginia: Great Ocean Publishers, 1997.

Jensen, Eric. *Brain-based Learning & Teaching*. Northriding, South Africa: Lead the Field Africa, 1995.

Jensen, Eric. *The Learning Brain*. Northriding, South Africa: Lead the Field Africa, 1994.

Promislow, Sharon. *Making the Brain Body Connection*. West Vancouver: Kinetic Publishing Corporation, 1998.

Sunbeck, Deborah. *Infinity Walk*. Torrence, CA: Jalmar Press, 1996.

Contact details

For more information on workshops and training in South Africa or to find a Brain Gym® consultant in your area – kindly contact:

The Brain Gym ConneXion
P O Box 44389
LINDEN
Johannesburg
2104
(011) 888-5434
braingymconneXion@worldonline.co.za

For more information on Brain Gym® workshops, training and publications worldwide, kindly contact:

The Educational Kinesiology Foundation
P O Box 3396
Ventura, CA 93006-3396
1-800-356-2109
http://www.braingym.com

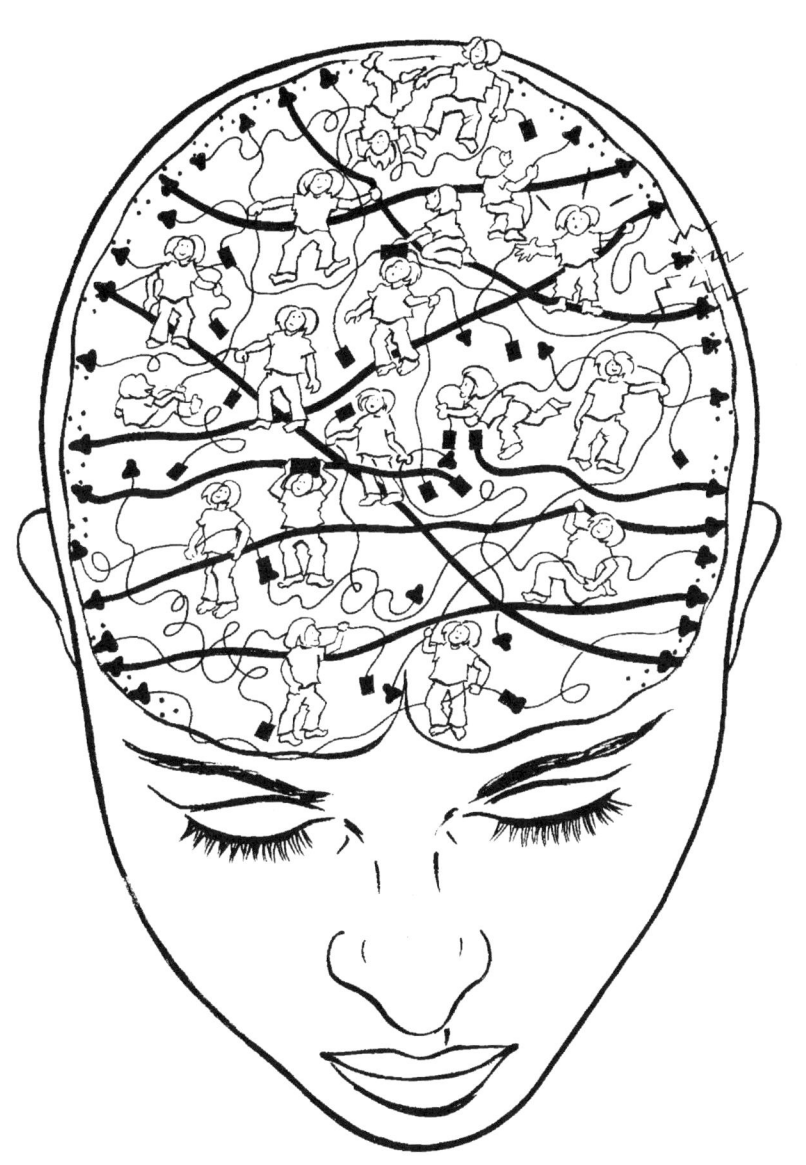